ANIMAL MAGNETISM AND THE LIFE ENERGY

Books by Jerome Eden

Animal Magnetism and the Life Energy
Planet in Trouble—The UFO Assault on Earth
Orgone Energy—The Answer to Atomic Suicide
Suffer the Children

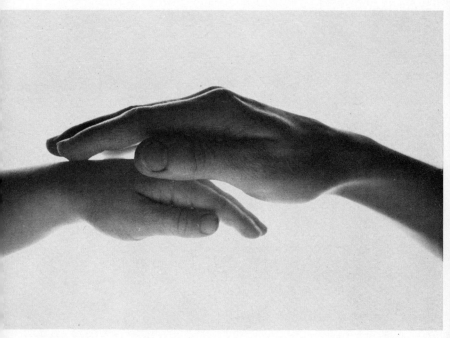

As the hands of the magnetiser gently stroke the subject, the Life Energy fields of both are excited to a degree where they will glow. *(Photo by Jim Laser.)*

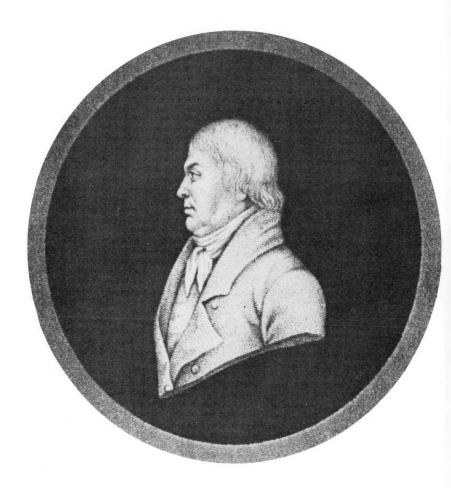

Franz Anton Mesmer, Doctor of Medicine (1734-1815).

Animal Magnetism and the Life Energy

Jerome Eden, M.A.,O.S.J.

Foreword by
BARBARA G. KOOPMAN, M.D., Ph.D.
Fellow, American College of Orgonomy

 EXPOSITION PRESS   HICKSVILLE, NEW YORK

ISBN 0-682-48045-2

Printed in the United States of America

This book is dedicated to the memory of two brilliant and courageous British physicians, Dr. John Elliotson and Dr. James Esdaile, whose devotion to Animal Magnetism, in the face of slander, ridicule, and much personal sacrifice, should not be forgotten.

"As God's purpose is to glorify the individual man or soul in the earth; so the highest purpose of an individual soul or entity is to glorify the Creative Energy, or God, in the earth."

Edgar Cayce
from *God's Other Door*

Contents

vii

Foreword

In this era of burning interest in psychic phenomena, Jerome Eden's volume on animal magnetism is a timely and exciting addition.

What is unfolding in our present-day society is an unsorted mélange of the occult, the mystical, the pseudo-scientific, the functional. People are forsaking the conventional pathways of religion and medicine in favor of body therapies, acupuncture, meditational disciplines, and a broad spectrum of psychic healing techniques.

Gaining in respectability and recognition are the trail-blazers of parapsychology detailed in such works as *Psychic Discoveries Behind the Iron Curtain*.[1] Even the pragmatic *Medical Economics*, a conventional journal widely read by physicians, offered a feature article highly lauding the work of Olga Worrall, a psychic healer of some renown.

It is most fitting that the works of Anton Mesmer should be spotlighted in this present setting. A great cloud of distortion has long surrounded these works. Zilborg,[2] for example, refers to Mesmer as "an unpleasant person, a psychological *sans-culotte*, a charlatanic contribution of Imperial Vienna to France on the eve of the Revolution." Though he later acknowledges the role of the "inveterate prejudice and standpat self-complacencies" of conventional science, he still devotes considerable space to the credentials of the committee of five appointed by the French Académie des Sciences to evaluate magnetism, a group which included Benjamin Franklin, "still sound of mind and limb and active." (Franklin, according to Mr. Eden's research, was ill

---

[1] By S. Ostrander and L. Schroeder, Prentice-Hall, 1970.
[2] *A History of Medical Psychology*, W. W. Norton, 1941.

and bedridden during the actual investigation.) Zilborg
then quotes the committee as the final authoritative word on
the subject: ". . . imagination without magnetism produces
convulsions and magnetism without imagination produces
nothing, [the members of the committee] have unanimously
concluded in regard to the question of the existence and usefulness of animal magnetic fluid that such fluid does not
exist and therefore cannot be useful . . ."

Mr. Eden helps to put magnetism in its proper place by
his insistence that much more than suggestion ("imagination") is at work here. Indeed, magnetism worked as well
on animals and preverbal children as it did on articulate
adults. Therefore to dismiss it as merely a form of hypnotic
suggestion is to overlook its deeper implications. Mr. Eden
has rightly, in my opinion, placed magnetism in the realm
of orgonotic phenomena, as discovered by Wilhelm Reich,
the founder of Orgonomy. What is common to both
Orgonomy and mesmerism is the use of the cosmic life
energy, which Reich called orgone, albeit the working techniques of the two modalities are quite different and should
not be confused.

As a practicing Orgonomist, I am intrigued by the red
thread running through all these energetically-based techniques—magnetism, acupuncture, psychic healing, vivaxis,
dowsing, hypnotism, biofeedback—in that all appear to be
working directly with cosmic energy and the orgone energy
field, or "aura," as it is termed in the esoteric literature.
Within this realm lie broad implications most tantalizing to
those of us who for years have been working with human
energy fields and observing them dance in color-tinged
swirls that change with the emotions and pulsatory state of
the organism.

Working independently in the 1930's and unknown to

each other, Reich[3] and H. S. Burr,[4] a Yale neurophysiologist, were the first to objectify the existence of an energy field around living organisms. Both used similar instrumentation, made possible by the advent of the triode tube. Reich later called the phenomenon the orgone energy field while Burr dubbed it the electrodynamic or L-field. Kilner,[5] a fully accredited British physician, considerably advanced the study of the human aura through techniques of objective visualization by means of dicyanin screens. Kilner was thus able to diagnose a multitude of disease states and even predict a patient's menstrual period four days in advance of its onset. All these fastidiously scientific works were ignored by the American medical profession. In recent years acupuncture has stirred some interest among medical men, though they invariably dismiss any energetic explanation as fanciful and opt for mechanistic "gate" theories.

Reich not only demonstrated the existence of the human energy field but also showed how it varied with alterations in affect. He demonstrated that pleasure and anxiety were at once functionally identical and antithetical: that is, both were the subjective perceptions of an objective energy flow in the organism—peripherally directed it was perceived as pleasure; centrally directed it was perceived as anxiety.[6]

Ravitz,[7] following in Burr's footsteps, replicated Reich's

---

[3]"Experimental Investigation of the Electrical Function of Sexuality and Anxiety" [Translation of 1937 monograph *Experimentelle Ergebnisse über die elektrische Funktion von Sexualität und Angst*], *Journal of Orgonomy*, Vol. 3, Nos. 1 and 2, 1969.

[4]"A Vacuum Tube Voltmeter for the Measurement of Bioelectrical Phenomena," *Yale Journal of Biology and Medicine*, Vol. 9, 1936-7.

[5]*The Human Aura*, University Books, 1965.

[6]Reich, W., *op. cit.*

[7]"History, Measurement and Applicability of the Electromagnetic Field in Health and Disease," *Annals of the New York Academy of Sciences*, Vol. 98, Art. 4, 1962.

observation of quantifiable fluctuations in field potential
varying with affective states. He further studied the field
reactions in altered states of consciousness and was able to
demonstrate a decreased amplitude in the post-induction
hypnotic state. He further found that changes in hypnotic
level could be detected immediately by voltage changes
which showed no relationship to classical criteria of hypnotic depth. Large voltage shifts were also noted when a
subject returned to the waking state. When following a
post-hypnotic suggestion, the subject's field potentials once
again reverted to the hypnotic pattern.

With such empirical investigations, the human aura—
once the domain of clairvoyants and occultists—has become
accessible to the man in the lab. Perhaps the most fascinating aspect of all is the sheer phenomenology of these energetic techniques—how do they actually work? Man is only
on the threshold of a breakthrough into the energetic realm;
he has attained great mastery over the secondary forms of
energy (the mechanical) but has as yet little insight into
the workings of cosmic primal energy. It was Reich's great
contribution to open up this primordial energy as an object
of scientific investigation for the functional thinker. Still
many questions remain unanswered.

If we turn to the various energetic—or, as I prefer to call
them—orgonotic modalities, certain intriguing facts emerge.
Take dowsing, for example. There are myriad devices used
for this purpose—angle wires, forked sticks, sophisticated
"aura meters," etc.—yet, to my knowledge, all must be held
within the aura of the dowser in order to get results. There
are some dowsers who need no devices at all but merely use
their own energy field; that is, the "antenna" appears to be
the dowser's field itself.

Even more fascinating is the specificity of the dowsing
process. To locate anything, one simply places a firm mental

image of the object in mind, be it water, gold, oil, or land mines. The instrument will then respond only to the concept of the object being sought. This leads to the idea, often expressed in the occult, that thoughts themselves are "things" and that every concept has an energetic blueprint that is peculiarly its own and exists objectively. I would postulate that the dowser uses his field to throw a charge into the "blueprint" which then resonates with the field of the sought-for object whenever he comes across it.

A related modality is acupuncture, which has profound effects upon the subject's field. These are easily seen by the trained observer in the form of an intense excitation and expansion. In my observation, if needles are applied to only one side of the body that side will show a marked expansion and charging up not evidenced by the other half of the body. From my subjective experience with a tonification treatment, I would guess that, along with the field excitation, a high degree of alpha brain wave activity is spontaneously evoked. In a relatively open subject, vegetative streamings, as described by Reich,[8] are readily felt. There is also a sensation of floating off the table. The state of relaxation is tremendous and there is no pain even with a profusion of needles *in situ*. In this modality, as in magnetism, polarity of the bodily energy is an important consideration.

The hypnotic process is equally intriguing and still remains an enigma. We have yet to explain how seeming verbal abstractions can induce changes on the physical plane. The problem is reminiscent of the dowsing rod's responding to a specific concept. We know from Ravitz that striking changes do occur in the field of the hypnotic subject, as registered in a decreased amplitude of the potential. I have personally observed a tremendous diffusion of the

---

[8]*Op. cit.*

energy field in subjects undergoing hypnosis (and also in meditation). I believe this diffused field state is a necessary concomitant of the hypnotic process. Perhaps it is partly due to the fact that any alterations of consciousness entailing marked diffusion of the field also break down ego boundaries. I would postulate that once the hypnotist's field is superimposed on the diffused field of the subject, the subject resonates with the conceptual blueprints of the hypnotist's field, rather than with his own field, which is non-intact.

However, I believe the hypnotic process is not entirely passive. The subject, in a sense, is really hypnotizing himself once he emotionally accepts the fact of hypnosis. The trigger in this case would be the superimposed field of the hypnotist. Autohypnosis and biofeedback training are somewhat different, though related. Here the subject provides his own conceptual blueprints as triggers. However, he must alter his state of consciousness first. In biofeedback subjects, a high degree of alpha brain wave activity has been well documented. I do not know what prevails in autohypnosis in this regard, but in hetereohypnosis subjects do not necessarily evoke a high degree of alpha activity, although they certainly show marked voltage changes in the energy field. We still have much to learn about these two parameters—field voltage changes and brain wave activity. Further knowledge of them might shed light on a very interesting difference Mr. Eden points out between hetereohypnosis and magnetism, namely, that in the former, the subject becomes increasingly susceptible to hypnotic suggestion while in the latter the subject loses his susceptibility to magnetism as he recovers his health.

It is of interest that one group of researchers, the Northwest Magnetics Research Society (Vivaxis) has serious reservations about the safety of hypnosis and allied modalities and feels the foreign fields superimposed in this manner upon a subject may adversely affect his mental and physical health.[9] They also have reservations about psychic healing in general for the same reason and have even evolved special techniques for clearing the aura of superimposed fields from foreign sources.

As for animal magnetism itself, I do believe it has a kinship with hypnosis. (I think Mr. Eden would agree.) However, Mr. Eden emphasizes the absence of verbal induction and the use of "physical" (energetic, really) techniques, such as hand passes. My personal guess is that a dual process unfolds: the charging up of the subject's energy field to a high pitch, the source of the charge being the fields of the magnetizer and his helpers (sometimes a chain of people backing him up), often augmented by devices similar to Reich's orac (orgone accumulator); the literal pulling out of stasis energy (what Reich termed DOR or deadly orgone radiation) from the organism by means of hand passes. Actual touching was not necessary and merely combing through the aura sufficed. Mr. Eden's observations about the operator's being grounded in water and the analogy to Reich's medical DOR-buster apparatus is well taken.

One would guess that the practitioners of magnetism must have been endowed with extremely powerful energy fields in order to be able to withstand the depletion of their charge and the absorption of toxic emanations from their patients.

There are countless examples of psychic healers one could cite—the occult literature abounds in them. Some, like the Kahunas, avoid depletion by what they regard as a process of channeling atmospheric energy into their sub-

---

[9]Nixon, F., *Born to Be Magnetic*, Vol. 2, Magnetic Publishers, British Columbia, 1973.

jects and directing it as if it had intelligence.[10] What must be common to all is a deep contact with and intuitive grasp of cosmic orgone energy functions. I believe that their procedures have nothing to do with intelligence—or, rather, that the intelligence resides not in the brain but in the total energy field of the practitioner and that this is the instrument at work if one will but open up and tune in. Most importantly, I feel that these processes can be removed from the realm of mysticism and form the new frontier of functional (as opposed to mechanistic) scientific investigation. This would require a certain openness of structure and capacity for health in the researchers themselves—no easy task in an armored society and polluted environment.

Jerome Eden is himself just such a seeker of knowledge. He has already given lavishly of his time and energy in the fight against man's despoiling of his planet.[11] He has rendered a further large service toward functional science by restoring Mesmer to his rightful place as a vital researcher into cosmic life energy.

BARBARA G. KOOPMAN, M.D., Ph.D.
Fellow, American College of Orgonomy

---

[10]Long, M. F., *The Secret Science Behind Miracles*, 5th ed., De Vorss and Co., Santa Monica, 1954.

[11]See *Orgone Energy*—The Answer to *Atomic Suicide*, Exposition Press, 1972.

Acknowledgments

Worldwide interest in psychic phenomena has refocused attention on one of the most controversial subjects ever presented to mankind—Animal Magnetism. Equally controversial was the originator of this subject, Dr. Franz Anton Mesmer, a heroic figure whose significant contributions to the understanding of "occult" phenomena deserve much greater attention than has hitherto been accorded.

While many books have been written about Mesmer himself, none presents a rounded picture of his theoretical formulations and actual therapeutic procedures. This book seeks to supply that information. To complete the picture, especially for the student of medicine, psychology, or psychic phenomena, more than a score of actual case histories are included here—cases ranging from epilepsy, insanity, and melancholia, to major surgery.

My own interest in Animal Magnetism (the terms "mesmerism" and "Animal Magnetism" are synonymous) began nearly twenty years ago with the discovery of little-known and untranslated works of Mesmer which were all but lost on the musty shelves of great libraries. I am convinced—and this work seeks to demonstrate—that Mesmer's work holds great promise in opening formerly mysterious realms dealing with ESP, mediumship, clairvoyance, and the occult generally. Of special importance here is the long and brilliant work of the late Dr. Wilhelm Reich, whose discovery of an objectifiable biological and cosmic energy places a firm foundation beneath Mesmer's theories and procedures. It is my hope also that this book will establish the true natural-scientific scope of mesmerism, and remove it from the obfuscating category of "hypnotism," where it has lain unproductive and neglected for nearly two hundred years.

My thanks go to the Association for Research and Enlightenment, Virginia Beach, Virginia, for permission to quote material from Edgar Cayce; and to Orgonomic Publications, Inc., New York, for allowing me to quote from my article, "The Emotional Plague Versus Animal Magnetism," which appeared in Vol. 1, No. 1 (1967) of *The Journal of Orgonomy*.

I take this opportunity to thank Mr. Harold Sherman, President of ESP Research Associates Foundation, for his helpful encouragement. And, finally, I wish to acknowledge the patient devotion my wife *Désirée* has given to this subject through the long years of preparation of this book.

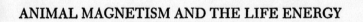
ANIMAL MAGNETISM AND THE LIFE ENERGY

1 *The Man and the Mystery*

While he lived he was the center of stormy controversy throughout Europe. Friends and colleagues hailed him as a "Savior of Mankind"; enemies railed against him as "Satan incarnate." Millions of words have been written, praising or condemning his ideas and his methods. Beggars and kings either cursed or idolized him; the wealthiest and the poorest sought his help. That man was Franz Anton Mesmer, Doctor of Medicine.

Today the world remembers Dr. Mesmer by such words as "mesmerize" and "mesmeric," which refer to the phenomenon called hypnotism. Many consider Mesmer as "the father of hypnotism," and thus one of the founders of modern-day psychology. As I shall show, however, none of these concepts of Mesmer's work is true. Mesmer never practiced hypnotism, which is essentially a *verbal and suggestive* technique whereby the subject is inducted into a light or deep sleep. Once the subject enters this sleeping state, the hypnotist gives verbal suggestions urging that the subject do this, or refrain from doing that.

Dr. Mesmer never employed the techniques of hypnotism. As we shall see, his theories and treatment of disease

3

are based upon *energetic* techniques that result in physiological changes in the human body. Psychologists and medical doctors who practice hypnosis today concede that, "for some strange reason," they cannot hypnotize patients with the degree of success attributed to Mesmer and his followers. This lack of success is usually blamed on faulty methods of hypnotic induction. Actually, the truth lies much deeper.

In the Foreword to his *Memoir of 1799,* Dr. Mesmer wrote: "I shall present a new and simple theory of diseases, of their arrestment and their development, and I shall substitute a method equally simple, general, *and found in nature,* for the uncertain principles which, up to the present time, have served as rules of medicine."

Here we get an inkling of the scope and magnitude of Mesmer's ideas. He will present a "new and simple theory of diseases." Hynotism cannot be considered to be a "new and simple theory of diseases." The phenomenon of hypnosis (the word itself comes from the Greek *hypnos,* meaning "sleep") has been known for thousands of years, long before Mesmer's announcements. Let us return to Mesmer's *Memoir* for some more light on this discussion: "By means of my theory I have attempted to explain the varied phenomena which have been classified as 'Somnambulism,' *phenomena which are nothing more than a critical development of certain diseases.* . . . I wish to affirm that all such strange manifestations are nothing more than *symptoms of critical periods* in certain nervous disorders."

We see from these quotations that Dr. Mesmer was thoroughly familiar with hypnotism and the hypnotic state, which he refers to as "somnambulism." He is cautious, however, in pointing out that somnambulism should not be confused with his methods and theories, because somnambulistic phenomena are nothing more than symptoms appearing in certain nervous disorders!

Now that we have some idea of the difference between Mesmer's method and hypnotism, let us see if we can determine what kind of actual therapeutic technique Mesmer is offering: "It is my hope that my theory will make accessible to cure those cases which were previously given up as hopelessly incurable. I am certain that the most dreadful conditions—such as madness, epilepsy, and the majority of convulsive disorders are merely aspects of illnesses of which medicine is still ignorant. . . . in brief, it is merely ignorance which prevents a cure."

What Dr. Mesmer is offering here is new hope for those suffering from the so-called incurable diseases. He is not naive enough nor fool enough to suggest that hypnotism (or "somnambulism") could *cure* such hitherto "incurable" maladies. It is therefore the purpose of this book to review the theories and actual practice of Dr. Mesmer, to survey many actual case histories, and to prove that what Dr. Mesmer did in fact discover was *a new and revolutionary method for the treatment and prevention of disease.* I further propose to show that Dr. Mesmer's postulates and theoretical assumptions, which underlie his actual medical procedures, have been fully vindicated in recent medical and cosmological discoveries in the United States. This is a large task indeed, and I beg the reader's patient indulgence. I have spent nearly twenty years in studying Dr. Mesmer's life and work. In the course of this time, I have had to translate virtually unknown and obscure manuscripts, written or dictated by Dr. Mesmer himself. I do believe, however, that the interested reader will come to realize the importance and significance of Dr. Mesmer's discoveries, discoveries which, after nearly two hundred years, are beginning to fulfill their promise of relief and mitigation of many of the "incurable" maladies which continue to plague humanity.

Before examining the actual theories and therapeutic procedures of Dr. Mesmer, let us review the life and scientific highlights of this "man of mystery." Franz Anton Mesmer was born May 23, 1734, in the Austrian village of Iznang on the shore of Lake Constance. The son of a gamekeeper, young Franz Anton grew up amid natural surroundings. His later scientific works indicate a deep love of nature, and he used many simple analogies to describe natural-scientific phenomena.

At first, the youthful Mesmer considered theology as a career, but after attending the Jesuit University at Dillingen in Bavaria, he decided against the religious life. He obtained a doctorate in philosophy and one in law before settling upon medicine as his life's work.

In 1766 he passed his medical examination at the University of Vienna with honors. Gerhard van Swieten, famous physician to the Imperial Court, signed Mesmer's diploma, which was awarded on the basis of the candidate's thesis, entitled "The Influence of the Planets Upon the Human Body."

Mesmer married the wealthy Widow von Posch in 1768. Their spacious home at Number 261 Landstrasse attracted notables from many lands, and Mesmer counted the Mozarts (both father and son) among his many friends. Indeed, Mesmer had become extremely proficient in playing the "glass harmonica," an instrument composed of finely blown glass goblets which were played by stroking them with moistened fingers. Interestingly enough, across the ocean Dr. Benjamin Franklin, who was to play such a crucial role in the fate of Mesmer's work, had also developed a passionate interest in the glass harmonica. Franklin actually mechanized the musical instrument so that the goblets could be rotated by a foot-actuated pulley and belt.

"Do you know," wrote Leopold Mozart to his wife in August 1773, "Herr von Mesmer plays . . . the harmonica unusually well? He is the only one in Vienna who has learnt it . . . Wolfgang too has played upon it. How I should like to have one!"

Thus, until Mesmer began to evidence a serious interest in what he was later to call "Animal Magnetism," he was a highly sought-after and respected member of Viennese cultural life. No one would deny his intelligence, his charm, and his generosity. He read widely and thoroughly and was well aware of the interesting experiments being performed with iron magnets.

It is quite likely that he was familiar with the deeds of such healers as Valentine Greatrakes, whose "miraculous" cures by the laying on of hands caused a great stir in England in the seventeenth century. He was also well aware of the work of Father Joseph Gassner, the Swabian priest whose "miracles" Mesmer later duplicated and explained on the basis of his own medical discoveries. And then there was Jean Baptiste van Helmont (1577-1644), a follower of Paracelsus, who taught that a "magnetic fluid" radiates from men and that it can be guided by their wills and influence the minds and bodies of others.

Paracelsus himself, a bombastic medical gadfly, roared at his medical colleagues: "A physician should be the *servant* of Nature—not her enemy! He should be able to guide and direct her in her struggle for life, and not throw, by his unreasonable influence, fresh obstacles in the way of recovery!" Such scathing directness did not endear Paracelsus to his medical brethren.

The Use of Magnets

In 1773, Mesmer had occasion to treat Franziska Oester-lein, age 29, with some iron magnets made by the Jesuit astronomer Father Maximillian Hell, who was then Professor of Astronomy at the University of Vienna. Father Hell believed that somehow the magnetic properties inherent in iron magnets could be directed to various parts of the human body if the magnets used were shaped to conform to the configuration of the organ or external anatomy over which they were placed.

"We found Fraulein Franzl in bed," wrote Leopold Mozart to his wife. "She is really very much emaciated, and if she has another illness of this kind, she will be done for!" After Mesmer applied his magnets for several hours to the woman's solar plexus and feet, she complained of "unusual currents" coursing through her body. Repeated applications of the magnets produced a "crisis," after which the patient felt much relieved.

When the malady gave way to his repeated treatments, Mesmer reported his findings to Father Hell, who immediately claimed that full credit belonged to the use of his magnets alone. Mesmer discovered, however, that the patient described the same "unusual currents" and displayed the same "critical symptoms" when the physician *passed his hands over the patient's body, without using the magnets!* Further experimentation convinced Mesmer that the magnets were merely "conductors of a subtle, tenuous fluid," which could act directly upon the patient's nervous system. He therefore dispensed with the use of magnets entirely.

In 1779, in order to dispel the false reports that sought to identify his work exclusively with the use of iron magnets, Mesmer published a brief history of his discovery in the *Memoir on the Discovery of Animal Magnetism* (1779).

Mesmer chose the term "Animal Magnetism" with great care. His experiments with many patients had demonstrated a form of "attraction and repulsion" analagous to what one finds in handling iron magnets. He wished to indicate a similarity between the "forces" operating in and around the human organism and those effective in iron magnetism. He declared that the living organism displayed a definite *polarity*, and that the same "substance" that operated within an iron magnet and that influenced the needle of a compass —this same "Universal Fluid" operated in *living organisms!* He chose the term "Animal Magnetism" to indicate two basic phenomena: first, that there is a definite similarity between the human organism and the iron magnet, in that they both obeyed natural law; and second, that the *"magnetism" of the living* was specifically "animal" (from the Latin word *anima,* meaning "soul"). Thus "Animal Magnetism" means "Soul Magnetism."

Instead of receiving the scientific interest and recognition he desired, Mesmer was stunned and bewildered by the amount of professional hatred and ridicule his work brought. The tide of scientific animosity grew in direct proportion to Mesmer's increasing ability to alleviate and cure the so-called "incurable" cases of his day. Even Dr. van Swieten and Dr. van Haen, who at first sent their most difficult cases to their former pupil, at length viewed Dr. Mesmer's successes with increasing alarm. Although Mesmer repeatedly invited many physicians and professors of science to witness his methods on intractable cases, few condescended to visit his treatment rooms. Most preferred to discuss his "weird and crazy" methods behind closed doors. Malicious gossip developed into whispering campaigns against "this young upstart."

Those who had been content to intrigue secretly against Mesmer now began to spread vicious rumors questioning his "morality." Official charges were brought against him by the Medical Faculty, and he was told to discontinue his "fraudulent practice" or face expulsion. Mesmer's patients were secretly interrogated: "Did Doctor Mesmer actually *touch* you? Did he stroke you? What else did he do?" The Austrian Committee to Sustain Morality was alerted, and Mesmer was confronted by the Chief of Police. In the face of slander and ridicule, with no chance to defend himself to his medical colleagues, Mesmer had no alternative but to leave Vienna and seek some other, "more enlightened climate."

Mesmer in Paris

Mesmer went briefly to Switzerland and then decided to try Paris, arriving there in February 1778. His wife, who was unsympathetic to his experiments with Animal Magnetism, did not accompany him. She was to die, about ten years later, of breast cancer.

The expatriated physician soon discovered that the malicious gossip and undermining that had poisoned the atmosphere in Austria had preceded him to France. Nevertheless, Dr. Charles Deslon, personal physician to the Count d'Artois (brother of Louis the sixteenth), attached himself to Mesmer as a willing pupil. On Deslon's insistence, Mesmer drafted an outline of his work that gave the general description of the attributes of the "Universal Fluid," the *agent* that, Mesmer believed, was responsible for all of the phenomena of Animal Magnetism. At a special assembly of the French medical fraternity, Deslon read Mesmer's "Twenty-Seven Propositions" and attempted to explain Animal Magnetism to his colleagues. The "Propositions" were rejected on September 18, 1780. Thereupon the Royal Society of Medicine decreed that any "doctor regent" who advocated or practiced

Animal Magnetism would be deprived of his diploma, and would thus forfeit the right to practice medicine.

The reaction of the French scientists was a duplication of what Mesmer had suffered in Vienna. Prior to the decision of the Royal Society, Mesmer had selected several severe cases, and taken these patients to his establishment at Creteil, six miles from Paris. He applied to the Royal Society of Medicine to examine and verify the diagnoses of these patients. The Society sent two physicians for that purpose; however, these gentlemen declined to make a formal report. The illnesses chosen (epilepsy, paralysis, blindness, and deafness) might, they said, "be faked."

Mesmer then applied to Vic d'Azyr, secretary of the Royal Society, asking permission to present his patients before the entire Society for certification as to the reality of their illnesses. "Men who doubt their ability to ascertain the truth of diseases," Mesmer wrote, "would doubt still more when requested to pronounce on their restoration to health." At the same time Mesmer enclosed certificates by independent members of the Society attesting to the genuineness of the disease of these patients. Nevertheless, Mesmer's application was refused and his certificates were returned unopened.

Again the tide of scientific animosity grew in proportion to Mesmer's successful treatments with Animal Magnetism. There was, for example, the famous case of Major Charles du Hussay, Major of Infantry and Knight of the Royal and Military Order of Saint Louis, who suffered from the results of typhus which he had contracted in the Indies. By his own admission, the Major was broken in mind and body, a physical wreck, having undergone every known form of therapy practiced by orthodox medicine. As a last resort, and without hope, he visited Dr. Mesmer. Major Hussay's statement follows:

After four years of useless experiments and the constant attendance of eminent physicians, among whom I can name several members of the Royal Society of Medicine in Paris, who personally know me and my case, I consented—as a last resort—to accept the proposition of Dr. Mesmer to try the proceedings of a method hitherto unknown. When I arrived at his establishment my head was constantly shaking, my neck was bent forward, my eyes were protruding from their sockets and greatly inflamed, my tongue was paralyzed, and it was with the utmost difficulty that I could speak. A perpetual and involuntary laugh distorted my mouth, my cheeks and nose were of a purple red, my respiration was very much embarrassed, and I suffered a constant pain between the shoulders. All my body trembled and I staggered when walking. In a word, my gait was that of an old drunkard, rather than that of a man of forty.

I know nothing of the means resorted to by Dr. Mesmer; but that which I can say with the greatest truth is that, without using any kind of drugs, or other remedy than "Animal Magnetism," as he calls it, he made me feel the most extraordinary sensations from head to foot. I experienced a crisis characterized by a cold so intense that it seemed to me that ice was coming out of my limbs. This was followed by a great heat, and a perspiration of a very fetid nature, and so abundant at times as to cause my mattress to be wet through.

The crisis lasted over a month. Since that time I have recovered and now, after four months, I stand erect and easy. My head is firm and upright, my tongue moves perfectly, and I speak as well as anyone. My nose and cheeks are natural, my color announces my age and good health; my respiration is free, my chest has expanded, and I feel no pain whatever. My limbs are steady and vigorous. I walk very quickly, without care and with ease. My digestion and appetite are excellent. In a word—I am perfectly free from all infirmities.

(signed) Ch. Du Hussay, etc.

Cases such as this one did not endear Mesmer to his fellow physicians, especially those who had pronounced Major Hussay, as well as others, "incurable."

Throughout his stay in France, Mesmer was avoided by the majority of the traditional scientific community. Despite the growing fame of his work, he was never permitted to demonstrate his method under controlled conditions before his fellow physicians. There were, however, a handful of courageous and dedicated scientists who viewed the "incredible phenomena" of Animal Magnetism, and who dedicated themselves to using this new therapy. These scientists and noblemen formed the Harmonic Society of France and invited Mesmer to teach the members his principles and procedures. One of the members, the Marquis de Lafayette, wrote to George Washington with glowing enthusiasm: "I know as much as ever a sorcerer knew!"

In general, however, silence or ridicule was the only response Mesmer received from his peers. The masses, on the other hand, flocked in droves to Mesmer's treatment rooms, along with the nobility who thronged the court of Marie Antoinette. Mesmer became the most discussed physician in France, and the more fashionable adopted Animal Magnetism as their newest pastime. Plays and musicales were produced, satirizing patients who "underwent crisis" and depicting Dr. Mesmer as some mysterious magician, with hat, cloak and wand, who presided over bizarre scenes designed to separate his clients from their money. Nothing was said of the fact that Dr. Mesmer often treated the impoverished without fees, feeding and housing them in his own home during prolonged periods of treatment.

Weary of the gossip, the constant harassment, and the undermining of his work, Mesmer decided to quit France. Mesmer's absence did not quell the gossip and intrigue against him and Animal Magnetism. Louis XVI was prevailed upon—in Mesmer's absence—to appoint a special Commission to sit in judgment of Animal Magnetism and render a report of its efficacy. Mesmer's absence, it was stated, was beneficial to a fair and impartial investigation, inasmuch as the commissioners would not be "unduly influenced by the presence of the discoverer." This would be exactly similar to asking the enemies of Madame Curie to present the facts regarding the discovery of radium "in Madame Curie's absence, because we do not wish to be unduly influenced by the lady's presence"!

Headed by Benjamin Franklin, who was visiting Paris at the time, the Commission included Lavoisier (the discoverer of oxygen) and Lavater (a chemist). In addition, there was Guillotin (advocate of the "humane" decapitator that bears his name), and Jean Sylvan Bailly, a botanist. Upon learning of the Commission's intentions, Mesmer wrote a furious letter to Franklin protesting the investigation on two basic counts: first, that Mesmer himself was not present; and second, that the Commission was to investigate the work of Dr. Charles Deslon, a former student of Mesmer *whom Mesmer had disavowed!* Mesmer affirmed that Charles Deslon was *not* practicing Animal Magnetism. As so often happens with "disciples" who suddenly "know more than their teacher," Dr. Deslon had discarded Mesmer's basic theoretical formulations concerning the existence of a "Universal Fluid" and was concentrating instead upon the somnambulistic phenomena "of the imagination."

Since it was a foregone conclusion that Animal Magnetism would be condemned, the actual "investigation" was merely a rubber-stamping process to officially destroy what had been privately ridiculed. Even before the Commission began its bogus investigation, the Royal Society of Medicine had gone on record as forbidding any physician to practice this therapy. Thus the Commission's final verdict was a surprise to no one.

In general, the Commission's voluminous Report denied the existence of any agent known as Animal Magnetism and claimed that all phenomena observed were "due to imagination and contact." Privately, a secret report was prepared for the King, in which the "immorality" of Animal

Magnetism was described, as well as the dangers inherent in a system that "denied the patient competent medical treatment."

An interesting comment on the Committee's Report was made by Dr. Joseph du Commun, an instructor at the United States Military Academy at West Point. In his book *Three Lectures on Animal Magnetism*, published in 1829, Dr. du Commun wrote:

> I cannot pass over in silence at this moment a circumstance most unfavorable in the United States to the cause of this discovery. Benjamin Franklin, the great Franklin, the honor of this country and the friend of France, was, on account of his great popularity and his known merit as a philosopher, appointed by the King of France one of the commissionaries, and he signed in that capacity the fatal report. To this unfortunate circumstance we must probably ascribe the difficulty this discovery has met with to find its way among you. Indeed his signature seemed to be a deadly stroke. Still, when we consider how it was obtained, its effects on our opinion must be modified. *Franklin was sick; he did not attend to any experiment.* . . . They presented the report, *to which he put his name while in bed, labouring under acute pains.* (Italics added.)
>
> All that we can infer from the case is that Franklin had a strong prejudice against Magnetism. I shall not expiate any more on that point, but leave to Franklin himself to apologize in his private memoirs: "We sometimes embrace an opinion which we think correct, but upon maturer reflection we change it for the very reverse."

It is true that Benjamin Franklin was in France at the time to engage the aid of the French Monarchy and to solicit friends for the troubled American Colonials. Nonetheless, a responsible "scientist" does not sign "reports" approving or disapproving a new discovery *in absentia!* Under Franklin's extremely influential signature, 60,000 copies of this Report were circulated throughout the world! This demonstrates an incredible effort in time and money to obliterate a "nonexistent discovery"! Where there is that much of a smoke screen, one would be wise to suspect "at least a little fire."

The effect of the Commission's Report was devastating and irreversible. Mesmer eventually retired from the social scene, secure in the knowledge that he had done his best for his discovery and for humanity. Returning to his beloved Lake Constance, he died on March 5, 1815, at the age of 81.

Principles of Animal Magnetism

Franz Anton Mesmer's discovery of Animal Magnetism is based upon his postulation of the existence of a "Universal Fluid." This is made crystal clear, as we shall see, in his "Twenty-Seven Propositions." Again, in Mesmer's *Memoir of 1799*, the theoretical assumption of a Universal Fluid forms the foundation of his entire theory and practice of Animal Magnetism.

All too often, those who investigated Mesmer's work were quick to dismiss as humbug his fundamental assumption of the existence of a "basic substance, so tenuous as to be able to penetrate all matter." And since Mesmer's discoveries coincided with the establishment of the science of electrical energy, many believed that Mesmer was simply confusing electrical phenomena with a "nonexistent Universal Fluid." This difficulty confronting Mesmer was compounded by the fact that he was never able to verify *objectively* the existence of his postulated Universal Fluid. "What is this strange Universal Fluid?" his detractors asked. "Can you touch it, see it, or measure its existence? And if you cannot touch it, or measure it in any way, then it simply does not exist!" Animal Magnetism had to wait nearly two hundred years before a twentieth-century scientist did scientifically verify the existence of such a "fluid."

Nonetheless, Mesmer did not merely take the existence

of such a Univeral Fluid on faith. He *did* offer evidence to verify its existence. For one thing, many of his patients, during the course of their therapy, reported actually *seeing* a grayish-blue "vapor" emanating from the body of the physician, particularly from his fingertips, eyes, and nose. Mesmer claimed that when he held his fingers over a glass of water, the Universal Fluid went from his fingers into the water. His patients said they actually could see the Universal Fluid filling the water glass. Again and again, Mesmer (as well as other physicians) demonstrated the curious effect that this so-called "magnetic water" had upon their patients—an effect that was totally absent in these same patients when they were given plain water.

Mesmer invented an apparatus that he called a "magnetic tub," which *accumulated* this Universal Fluid and made it available to his patients. He believed that the Universal Fluid existed everywhere in the atmosphere, that it was responsible for the "intension and remission" of natural phenomena—of seasonal cycles, tides, the "respiration" of the ocean, animal and bird migrations. It was this Universal Fluid that determined the health or illness of an individual. Blockage of the body's Universal Fluid caused "stagnation" and eventual illness. Treatment, therefore, consisted in overcoming the blockage of Universal Fluid. This could be accomplished either by "adding" more Universal Fluid to the ailing person or by removing the blockages.

Let us picture a free-flowing stream (the Universal Fluid) that is suddenly blocked by a fallen tree. In the body, according to Mesmer, such a blockage occurs through chronic muscular contractions, through chronic muscular expansions, or through the inability of certain muscular tissue to expand or contract at all. The blockage may either be removed directly, by working upon the "tree," or by *increasing* the stream-flow (Universal Fluid) until there is enough Fluid to force the blockage to give way. A "crisis" always accompanies such a breakthrough, Mesmer maintained. And without a sufficient crisis, no effective cure can be accomplished.

If Mesmer's postulation of a Universal Fluid was humbug —as his detractors maintained—then let it be recorded that Sir Robert Boyle (1627-1691), founder of the Academy of London, must have been bitten by the same humbug, inasmuch as he too believed in the existence of the Universal Fluid that enabled individuals "to exercise an action upon each other."

The Baron Charles von Reichenbach, famed German chemist, must also have succumbed to the bite of this humbug. This illustrious man, some of whose experiments appear in this book, spent many years documenting just such a Universal Fluid, which he termed "Od," or the "Odic force."

Let it also be noted that the eminent physician John Elliotson, M.D., FRS, who was the first to introduce the use of the stethoscope to British physicians, was also a firm believer in the existence of the Universal Fluid. Dr. Elliotson was selected to deliver the nineteenth Herveian Oration in London—a singular honor accorded to the most outstanding scientist each year. Dr. Elliotson's subject for that oration, delivered on June 27, 1846, was "Mesmerism." His conviction of the truth and efficacy of Animal Magnetism and the existence of a Universal Fluid cost him his position as senior physician and professor at the North London Hospital. Thomas Wakley, editor of the *Lancet,* savagely castigated Elliotson for his "mesmeric humbug." The practice of Animal Magnetism was thereupon prohibited at North London Hospital, whereupon Dr. Elliotson immediately resigned, continuing the practice of Animal Magnetism until his death in 1868.

From April 1843 to December 1855, Elliotson edited and published a journal called *The Zoist: A Journal of Cerebral*

Physiology and Mesmerism and Their Application to Human Welfare. As a quarterly publication, *The Zoist* presented scores of case histories by physicians and others practicing Mesmerism throughout the world, and most of the cases presented in this book first appeared in *The Zoist.* Among the surgical cases presented are those of Dr. James Esdaile (1808-1859), a brilliant British surgeon who employed Animal Magnetism as the sole anesthetic in more than 300 major surgical operations that were performed in India. So grateful was the Indian Government that it erected for Esdaile the Mesmeric Hospital of Calcutta. Dr. Esdaile utilized Animal Magnetism in many nonsurgical cases, and suffered insults and defamation for his pioneering efforts. His magnificent book *Mesmerism in India* was republished in 1957 under the misleading title *Hypnotism in Medicine and Surgery.*

The Bioenergetic Basis of Animal Magnetism

I feel obliged to record that my own interest in Animal Magnetism coincided with my knowledge and duplication of some of the experiments of the late Dr. Wilhelm Reich. Briefly, Reich discovered what he termed "orgone" energy —the primordial, mass-free, pre-atomic energy of our planet, the same energy that operates in the living organism as the biological Life Energy. Years of my own personal verification of Reich's findings convinced me that Reich was absolutely correct in his discovery of a Cosmic Life Energy (see my book, *Orgone Energy—The Answer to Atomic Suicide,* Exposition Press, New York, 1972).

It was my knowledge of orgone energy that enabled me to touch and comprehend the discoveries of Franz Anton Mesmer. Thus it was that in the twentieth century, Wilhelm Reich—without knowing of the work of Mesmer—substantiated Mesmer's claims of the existence of a Universal Fluid.

The scientific researcher and serious student would be strongly advised, therefore, to study the discoveries of Reich in order to understand the functional laws governing this biological energy. *The credit for the actual scientific discovery and scientific verification of a Cosmic Life Energy belongs solely and exclusively to Wilhelm Reich.* I believe that Mesmer's expressed hope that "some talent, better understood than mine. . . . might go further than I," was completely fulfilled in the vital discovery of orgone energy by Wilhelm Reich.

The reaction to Reich's work in the twentieth century was identical in every respect to what Mesmer suffered nearly two hundred years before. Reich was hounded from country to country. All kinds of distorted claims were made for and against his work. In defense of his work, Reich was imprisoned in a United States federal penitentiary, where he died in 1957.

But, to return to our review of Animal Magnetism: neither unjustified condemnation nor unjustified credulity is grounds enough to favor the rational scientific examination of Mesmer's claims. I do not present Animal Magnetism either as a panacea or a parlor game, nor do I make any claims for its therapeutic effectiveness. What I do maintain, however, is that Dr. Mesmer's discovery of Animal Magnetism can only be properly judged according to the principles and procedures laid down by Dr. Mesmer, and *not* according to the principles and procedures of Charles Deslon or advocates of "hypnotism." If one is to judge Animal Magnetism, it would seem reasonable to expect that one would return to Mesmer's original principles and procedures. Unfortunately, this has not been the situation in the past. Almost without exception, every single reference work that lists Animal Magnetism or Franz Anton Mesmer confuses Animal Magnetism with hypnotism.

It was Mesmer's basic contention that Animal Magnetism is both a theory and a method of treating and preventing disease. As we shall see again and again, treatment by Animal Magnetism is based upon *physical contact*—that is, *touch*. The hands of the therapist are used in making "passes" over the patient's body in specific ways. Treatment may take anywhere from a few short moments to daily hour-long sessions lasting months, and even years. No suggestions of any kind—either verbal or otherwise—are required; and whether the patient falls asleep or remains fully awake is immaterial.

Hypnotism, on the other hand, is not of itself a therapeutic agent, and no responsible hypnotist would ever claim it as such. Furthermore, no hypnotist would claim that he could beneficially treat the diseased or bruised legs of animals—although such cases have been successfully treated by Animal Magnetism, as we shall see. In addition, whereas the hypnotized subject becomes increasingly susceptible to the hypnotic state with every "treatment," Animal Magnetism becomes increasingly *ineffectual* as the patient approaches health. In fact, Mesmer's criterion of health is *the inability of the patient to be further affected by Animal Magnetism!*

It is not so much that I object to the mislabeling of Animal Magnetism as "hypnotism" on the grounds of mere semantics, but rather that such mislabeling tends to remove Animal Magnetism from the category of the energetic and physiological and erroneously classifies it as "metaphysics," incapable of scientific inquiry and rational development.

In 1957 I brought out the first English translation of Mesmer's *Memoir of 1799*, followed in 1958 by the *Maxims on Animal Magnetism*. The *Memoir of 1799* contains Mesmer's attempt to develop a theoretical basis for his discovery of Animal Magnetism. Not only is the *Memoir* an extremely difficult book to read, but also it lacks the scientific data required to formulate any accurate theoretical basis. Nevertheless, Mesmer made a noble effort in this direction. I have extracted some of the more significant portions of the *Memoir* for presentation in this work. The *Maxims,* however, is reproduced in its entirety at the end of this book.

In 1967 my article "Emotional Plague versus Animal Magnetism" appeared in the first issue of *The Journal of Orgonomy,* a scientific journal of the highest quality published semiannually by Orgonomic Publications, Inc., Box 565, Ansonia Station, New York, N.Y. 10023. It is suggested that the serious student subscribe to this journal for current findings and elaborations on the basic discoveries of Dr. Wilhelm Reich.

As I have stated elsewhere, it was my knowledge of the discoveries of Reich that enabled me to make contact with and grasp the significance of Mesmer's discoveries made some two centuries earlier. I consider myself, therefore, simply as a functional guide whose work in the present context consists in pointing out some of the major connections between Mesmer's discoveries and Reich's objectively verified findings with respect to the latter's work on the Life Energy (orgone energy) of man and his universe.

Since I began to focus attention on Mesmer's neglected work about twenty years ago, there have been some researchers and writers in science and metaphysics who have, out of ignorance or deliberate distortion, attempted to minimize Reich's priorities by stating that researchers before Reich actually discovered the Life Energy. Such writers have used Mesmer as an example of one who actually "discovered" the biological Life Energy and used it years before Reich's interests led him into this field. As I stated in "Emotional Plague versus Animal Magnetism":

Regardless of how close Mesmer's principles and practice approach functional law, and although Franz Anton Mesmer did, in effect, use the cosmic and biological orgone energy, *he cannot be credited with the factual, objectively verifiable discovery of the orgone.* That honor belongs solely to Wilhelm Reich. One may postulate the existence of a primordial, cosmic energy; one may even use it practically and beneficially (as a mother does whenever she strokes her child's bruised limb), but postulation and use alone do not constitute a scientific discovery.

The Universal Fluid Is Orgone Energy

The "Universal Fluid" postulated by Mesmer (as presented in his "Twenty-Seven Propositions," and in his *Memoir* and *Maxims*) is in fact cosmic orgone energy, which, operating in the living organism, is *the* Life Energy, per se, first objectively verified by Reich between 1936 and 1940. Of this there can be no doubt whatsoever.

Readers of my book *Orgone Energy* will recall that the orgone was discovered by Reich in the atmosphere and in man, that its basic color is blue or bluish gray, that it penetrates *all* substances, that it can be accumulated in Reich's Orgone Energy Accumulator (Mesmer's *baquet*), and that it has an "opposing" energy variant that Reich named "DOR," or *D*eadly *OR*gone energy, a highly toxic, radioactive substance that is literally deadly to the living. In 1944 Reich was successful in taking an X-ray photograph of the excited orgone-energy field between the palms of two hands, which he published in his *Orgone Energy Bulletin* in 1948. Reich scientifically verified the existence of orgone energy visually, thermically, electroscopically, microscopically, by Geiger counter, by Orgone Energy Field Meter, and with various other inventions, such as the "DOR-Buster" or "Cloudbuster." The DOR-Buster, a device for removing biologically stale, exhausted and harmful DOR from the body, appears similar to Mesmer's invention of the "wet baquet." Further similarities in the work of Mesmer and Reich can be seen in Mesmer's postulations regarding the role played by muscular blockage in obstructing the flow of the body's "universal fluid" and Reich's discovery of muscular "armoring"—that is, chronic muscular rigidities which block the free flow of orgone energy in the body. (See Reich's *Character Analysis,* and Dr. Elsworth F. Baker's *Man in the Trap,* Macmillan, 1967.)

Nevertheless, Mesmer was not a functional thinker: he was a mechanist. The fact that he grasped and tenaciously affirmed a belief in a universal *fluidum,* that he explored the effects of this "subtle agent" in man and his universe, places Mesmer in a unique position in the history of science, leading up to and finally fulfilled in Reich's brilliant discovery of the Life Energy in the twentieth century. There was, however, as Reich pointed out, only one correct avenue of approach to this magnificent discovery—*the orgastic plasma convulsion.* (See Reich's *The Function of the Orgasm.*) This was Reich's (and science's) single most important discovery. Without it, man could gain no access to the objectification of the Life Energy and a comprehension of its laws. The discovery of the function of the orgasm was to prove the one and only cornerstone upon which a true Science of Life could be built. Without such knowledge, Mesmer could not comprehend the *living,* could not objectify his "Universal Fluid," and was unable to formulate a functional thought technique to develop his discoveries further.

On the other hand, the processes of Animal Magnetism produced some amazing phenomena. The case histories recorded here (as well as hundreds of others) defy explanation in terms of classical or orthodox medicine and science. Let us see if we can open an approach to an understanding of Animal Magnetic phenomena on the basis of orgonomic knowledge.

Reich's work shows that two organisms, which are basically two separate orgone energy systems, can mutually excite each other as they approach one another. When Mesmer made "passes" with his hands over the body of a patient, it is clear that the energy field from his palms and fingertips was interacting with the weaker energy field of the sick person. Following Reich's "orgonomic potential," the biological energy would flow from the weaker system (the patient) to the stronger system (the doctor). As peripheral energy flowed out of the patient, he might fall asleep, because of the lowering of his own energy level. Also, it can be assumed that the patient undergoing Animal Magnetism lost some of his DOR as well. (One researcher noted that on occasion Mesmer would make passes while placing one foot into a tub of water. Hence, his own body was acting as a DOR-Buster,* grounding the DOR into the water bucket.)

As the passes were continued, hour after hour, day after day—sometimes for months, and longer—we can assume that the weaker energy field of the patient was being excited and strengthened and that fresh energy was reaching the biological core. As the patient's energy level increased, such an increase in bioenergy now came into contact with the chronic muscular armoring (the character structure) of the individual. This would explain the "crisis" (energetic breakthroughs) which Mesmer claimed must occur in order for any malady to be cured.

So, in order to experience a crisis, the patient must first build up a sufficient energy reservoir. This was accomplished

---

*A full description of the Reich DOR-Buster appears in my book, *Planet in Trouble* (Exposition Press, 1973).

via the passes performed by the physician, as well as by the close proximity of the physician's total energy field and its influence upon the sick person. The energy mobility as well as the energy level of the physician himself would therefore be of great importance in Mesmer's method. It should be noted that Reich pointed out in his book *The Murder of Christ* that certain people, like Christ, had an energy field strong enough to expand the fields of those they touched. Repeated bioenergetic excitation leads to *expansion*. And the "attractiveness" of highly "magnetic" persons is due to this high level of Life Energy.

Mesmer pointed out that the "seat" of all sensations lies in the area of the solar plexus, the "common sensorium," from which arise all of man's sensory organs. Reich often wrote of the "basic orgonotic sense." During treatment with Animal Magnetism, as peripheral biological energy is withdrawn, energy at the core is strengthened. The continual weakening of peripheral energy and simultaneous increase in core energy provide the reason for somnambulistic behavior, wherein the patient is both "asleep and awake" at the same time. As the core energy continued to increase, the patient was able to *make contact directly with the surrounding "world"!*

In the *nonliving* state, cosmic primordial energy is "in contact" with all cosmic primordial energy. When energy is excited in one area of the universe, such excitations, like ripples on a lake, are conveyed throughout the energy continuum. Human beings are, in a sense, "living tuning forks." Vibrations emanating from one are conveyed to all, but only those capable of the same vibrational frequency appear to respond. Past, present, and future, as Mesmer indicated in his *Memoir* are merely "points of view" as seen by any observer in contact with the "stream of life." If we look "upstream" we see the future; what moves before us is the present; and "downstream" is the past.

The "Invisible Fire"

Mesmer's patients often made mention of being able to see the "universal fluid" streaming off the doctor's fingertips, from his eyes, eyebrows, hair and nose. The descriptions of this Life Energy can refer to nothing less than Reich's orgone energy, the same energy described by many mystics as the human aura and employed for centuries by many religious groups in the "laying on of hands." Man is indeed quickened, enlivened by this Life Energy, which is responsible for maintaining the body's healthy condition and for restoring the health of the sick organism.

It is most interesting, and saddening, to realize that most civilized people today are unable to see this scintillating, constantly moving cosmic energy that is "right before our eyes." Reich showed that the inability to see the orgone is a result of chronic muscular rigidities, especially in the ocular area, which prevent immediate *contact* with the Life Energy. To the extent that such muscular "armor" is mobilized, the ability to actually see the orgone energy is restored. The question therefore arises as to why certain sick people, particularly those classified by Mesmer as suffering from "nervous irritability," could so easily perceive this "invisible fire" while undergoing treatment by Animal Magnetism. It is precisely here that researchers may find a doorway to the mysteries of clairvoyance, clairaudience, and all other phenomena commonly subsumed under the label "extrasensory perception," or ESP. As it is impossible to perceive anything "outside of" or "apart from" one's sensory apparatus, the term "extrasensory perception" is as erroneous as it is misleading. As

Mesmer indicated, what is involved here is a "tuning" or "focusing" of the sensory apparatus, similar to the way in which we focus a microscope or telescope.

I am convinced that serious scientific research into the "invisible fire" of orgone energy will prove of great benefit to the entire field of "psychic research," another misleading term, which considers "the mind" per se the "supreme" force of the living. As Reich pointed out time and again, the living functions beautifully long before the development of a brain. It is characteristic of mystical thinkers to place primary importance on an organ of man that is merely a complex relaying station. Anyone who undergoes psychiatric orgone therapy soon realizes that the body functions in accordance with the movement or blockage of its basic Life Energy— either as a harmonious unit or as an unharmonious, fragmented, that is, "armored," organism. One's memories and conscious awareness are as much a function of one's genital organs, thoracic and neck musculature as they are of one's brain. In the healthy person, the body is a functional unit: We love *wholly*, we work *wholly*, we concentrate on any task *wholly*. As the late Dr. Oscar Tropp once pointed out, the original definition of the word "health" is synonymous with "wholeness." There is simply no such thing as a "healthy mind" in an otherwise armored or unhealthy body.

But, to return to our consideration of the "invisible fire," the Life Energy of the human organism—there is another side to this "fire," a deadly, dangerous side that did not exist in the eighteenth and nineteenth centuries. I refer now to atomic or nuclear energy. It is most significant that the discoveries of orgone energy and nuclear energy were made almost simultaneously, as if mankind were being given a choice between crucial pathways to either Life or Death. Since I dealt with the subject of nuclear contamination of our planetary and biological Life Energy at great length in my book *Orgone Energy—The Answer to Atomic Suicide,* I shall only comment briefly here.

The contamination of the Life Energy by vast amounts of nuclear-energy uses on Earth is changing the benign and beneficent orgone energy into an irritating and highly excited form of energy called "oranur" by Wilhelm Reich. When harmful types of *secondary* energies (that is, energies derived *from* the primordial, mass-free, pre-atomic orgone energy) interact with orgone energy, the result is often extremely dangerous to the living. Besides nuclear energy production and use, additional irritating agents are high-voltage electricity, noxious chemicals and gases, TV sets, and ordinary fluorescent and neon lights. The existence of such "antagonistic" energy sources must always be kept in mind by those doing research on the Life Energy. Reich found that his Orgone Energy Accumulator, for example, would not function properly in the vicinity of the above-mentioned, secondary-energy sources, especially fluorescent lights. Many sensitive people find that their ability to function in such contaminated atmospheres is sharply curtailed.

As reported in the December 30, 1973 issue of *The National Enquirer,* Dr. John Ott, photobiologist, of the Department of Biology, University of South Florida, Tampa, Florida, stated that his experiments with fluorescent lights "strongly indicate that fluorescent lighting has a harmful effect on everyone who is subjected to it. . . . They become nervous, irritable and hyperactive." Dr. Ott further stated: "These lights give off soft X-rays, similar to color TV sets."

When we realize that millions of people, especially our most sensitive schoolchildren, are subjected to these gratuitous X-rays for many hours every day, is it any wonder that the health of civilized man is so rapidly declining?

Only by studying the functions of the Life Energy in man and his universe will we gain a firm and rational understanding of that which is "good" or "evil" with respect to our God-given Life Energy. All matter and all life are derived from the limitless cosmic orgone energy within which man and his universe are immersed. If man continues to contaminate the very *Source of Life,* then everything which arises from that source must inevitably partake of such contamination.

As the formerly clean and benign Life Energy is continually being corrupted by deadly secondary energies, we see the remarkable increase and attraction toward cults of darkness and evil, the preoccupation with Satanism and "possession." Evil men are in truth "possessed"—not by a mystical, demonic "creature," but rather by a Life Energy that has become stagnant and noxious (DOR). Thus, man's age-old mystical beliefs in God and Devil, good and evil, sin and love, and the conversion of the one into its opposite—all are beginning to be understood on the basis of Reich's magnificent discovery of orgone energy, the Life Energy.

The Life Energy is the "Fire of Life." Nuclear energy is the "Fire of Death." The one creates; the other can only destroy. The choice for humanity will be decisive.

2 *Principles and Procedures*

The Twenty-Seven Propositions of F. A. Mesmer

1. There exists a reciprocal influence between the heavenly bodies, the earth, and all animated bodies.

2. A fluid, universally diffused and so continuous as not to permit any vacuum, and the subtlety of which does not allow of any comparison, and which is capable of receiving, propagating, and communicating all impulses, is the vehicle of that influence.

3. This reciprocal action is governed by mechanical laws which are not known at present.

4. Alternating effects arise from this action—effects that may be considered as an ebb and flow.

5. This ebb and flow is more or less general, particular, or composite, according to the nature of the causes that determine it.

6. It is by this action—universally present in Nature—that active relations are established between the heavenly bodies, the earth, and its constituent parts.

7. The properties of matter and of organized bodies depend upon this action.

31

8. The living organism experiences the alternating effects of the Universal Fluid, which insinuates itself into the substance of the nervous system and *directly affects* the nervous system.

9. Properties similar to those of the iron magnet are found in the human body: different and opposite poles can be distinguished, which can be excited, changed, destroyed, or reinforced—even the phenomena of attraction and repulsion are observed in the living organism.

10. The property of the living organism which makes it susceptible to the influence of the heavenly bodies, and to the reciprocal action of those that surround it, has led me (from its analogy with the magnet) to call it "Animal Magnetism."

11. The action and power of Animal Magnetism can be communicated to other bodies, both animate and inanimate—both are more or less susceptible to it.

12. This action and power can be reinforced and propagated by the same bodies.

13. The flow of a material whose substance penetrates all bodies—without apparently losing its activity—can be observed experimentally.

14. The action of this Universal Fluid can occur at a great distance, without the aid of any intermediary body.

15. The Universal Fluid is augmented and reflected by mirrors, like light.

16. It is communicated, propagated and augmented by sound.

17. Its magnetic force can be accumulated, concentrated, and transported.

18. I have said that living bodies are not equally susceptible. There are some—though this is very rare—who have *an op-*

posite property, so that their mere presence destroys all the effects of this magnetism in other bodies.*

19. The opposite property also penetrates other bodies. It can be communicated, propagated, accumulated, concentrated, and transported, reflected in mirrors, and propagated by sound—which shows that it is not a mere privation, but a positive opposing influence.

20. The magnet, whether natural or artificial, is, like other bodies, susceptible of Animal Magnetism, and even of the opposing force, without in either case its action on the iron needle undergoing any alteration—which proves that the principle of Animal Magnetism differs essentially from magnetism of the mineral kind.

21. This system will furnish new ideas about the nature of fire and light and enlighten us with respect to the theory of attraction, of ebb and flow, of the magnet, and of electricity.

22. It will show that the magnet and artificial electricity have an effect on maladies similar to that of several other natural agents; and if some useful effects have come from their employment they are due to Animal Magnetism.

23. It will be established from the facts, according to the rules which I will set forth, that Animal Magnetism will cure, immediately, all diseases of the nerves, and, mediately, all other diseases.

24. Animal Magnetism provides the physician an insight into the use of drugs; he can improve their action and can bring on and direct beneficial crises, so as to make himself their master.

25. In communicating my method, I will demonstrate,

---

*The discovery of orgone energy and its deadly variant, DOR, shed much light on this assertion by Dr. Mesmer. As the antithesis of cosmic orgone energy, DOR does indeed "nullify" the orgone.

through a new theory of disease, the universal utility of the principle which I bring to bear against illnesses.

26. With this knowledge, the physician may judge with certainty the origin, nature, and progress of diseases, even the most complicated. He will check their advance, and will succeed in curing them without ever exposing the patient to dangerous effects or unfortunate consequences, whatever be the patient's age, temperament, or sex. Even women in pregnancy and childbirth will enjoy the same advantage.

27. Finally, my doctrine will place the physician in a position to judge accurately the degree of health of each person, and to preserve him from diseases to which he might be exposed. The healing art will thus attain to the utmost perfection.

These are the "Twenty-Seven Propositions" of Dr. Mesmer, which form the basis for his theory and practice of Animal Magnetism. Again and again we see his reference to the Universal Fluid—to its "ebb and flow," its ability to "penetrate everything." What Mesmer was in fact seeking was the discovery of a specific *biological energy*, the orgone energy, verified in more than thirty years of work in the twentieth century by Wilhelm Reich. Mesmer believed (and Reich proved) that we are all immersed in this "ocean of energy," that its correct application could improve health and reverse disease processes. The question then arises, How did Mesmer actually employ his Universal Fluid in the treatment of his patients? We must turn to his *Maxims on Animal Magnetism* for such information.

The *Maxims on Animal Magnetism* (actually a series of "aphorisms") were given by Mesmer in a course of lectures to interested physicians and students. Dr. Caullet de Veaumorel, who attended these lectures, wrote them down and published them in 1785 in a volume entitled *Aphorismes*. I brought out the first English translation of the *Maxims on Animal Magnetism* in 1958. As the *Maxims* are somewhat cryptic and make the strongest demands upon the reader, I shall present only the most pertinent ones here completely, and the remainder in synoptic form. The *Maxims* are numbered consecutively from 1 to 344. Those desiring more information are referred to my complete translation at the end of this book.

Principles

This first section of the *Maxims* consists of a review of Mesmer's principles. Here he attempts to explain the creation of "matter and motion," and from this the creation of more complex material substances. He refers to a "primary matter," that is, the Universal Fluid (Reich's orgone), stating that "the cessation of movement in matter produces solidity." Reich held that the creation of matter was the result of the superimposition of two orgone energy streams (see Reich's *Cosmic Superimposition*).

M44 (Maxim 44) states: "If we suppose a current which insinuates itself into a body, dividing itself into an infinite number of small currents . . . we call these subdivisions *streams*." Thus, according to Mesmer, man is immersed in an ocean of fluid (Cosmic energy); this fluid penetrates all interstices, because it is the "most tenuous, subtle substance of our atmosphere." M44 continues this thought: "The interstices or masses remain permeable to the currents or streams of the subtle substance." And, again, in M47: "All bodies submerged in this fluid are obedient to the movement of the fluid."

Sections Two and Three of the *Maxims* take up a discussion and consideration of cohesion and elasticity, while Section Four considers the phenomenon of "gravity." It is in Section Eight, "On Man," that Mesmer leaves the realms of cosmology and speculative physics and focuses upon the human being. Here he considers the question of "health." *When can we consider a person healthy?* "Man is in a condition of health when all parts of which he is composed are able to exercise the functions for which they were destined. If perfect order rules all of his functions, one calls this state the state of harmony" (M146 and 147). "Sickness is the opposite state—that is, one wherein harmony is disturbed" (M148). "The *remedy* is that which reestablishes the order or harmony which has been disturbed" (M152).

"Man, being continuously surrounded by universal and individual currents, is affected by them; the movement of the Universal Fluid becomes modified by the various structures of his parts, and the Universal Fluid becomes *tonic*. In this tonic state the Universal Fluid follows the continuity of the body and moves toward the most prominent parts" (M160).

Amplifying this discussion of the "flow" of biological energy within and without the human organism, Mesmer states: "From these prominences or extremities, the tonic currents flow away and rejoin the atmospheric currents. This occurs more readily *when a body capable of receiving or conveying them is placed in opposition to such extremities.* When this occurs, the currents become restricted into a point and their speed is increased." In other words, Mesmer is saying that the *extremities* or "prominences" of the human body are the best conductors ("receivers or conveyors") of the currents of biological energy—particularly the eyes, nose, chin, and most especially the hands and feet.

But what about an actual "polarity" of the body, which, according to Mesmer, "is analogous to the magnet"? He declares, "The points of outlet or entrance of tonic currents are what we call *poles*" (M162).

Section Nine of the *Maxims* deals with "sensations." How is it that man perceives anything? The "senses," he states, are merely "extensions" of a basic sensory apparatus, which Reich later described as the "first orgonotic sense," located in the region of the solar plexus. This throws light on such phenomena as people who "read" with their *palms* or with a book placed over their solar plexus; or others who can "see" through blindfolds, or who can "sense" colors through their fingertips.

Maxim 184 is particularly noteworthy: "It is very likely. . . . that we are endowed with an internal sense which is in communication with the entire universe. With it we are able to understand the possibility of presentiments." Those psychics and "sensitives" who are "in touch" with the biological and cosmic orgone energy to a high degree are thus able to "know" events at great distances. Mesmer compared such "sensitives" to a person standing upon a high cliff overlooking a river. "Upstream" from the observer constitutes the "future"; downstream constitutes the "past." The "stream" is the cosmic orgone energy in which we are all immersed.

Section Eleven of the *Maxims* discusses sickness. Here Mesmer makes a sharp distinction between *symptomatic symptoms* and *critical symptoms*. Effects produced by the cause of any disease are termed "symptomatic symptoms." If, on the contrary, "these effects are the efforts of nature *to overcome* the causes of the malady and to destroy such causes and restore harmony, we call them *critical symptoms*" (M206). The distinction between critical and symptomatic symtoms is important because, "In practice we must distinguish carefully between them, in order to prevent or arrest the one and promote the other" (M207).

Maxim 210 gives us again Mesmer's criterion for cure and

health: "*A body in harmony is insensible to the effects of Magnetism, since the proportion of the established harmony cannot be changed by the application of a uniform and general action.* On the other hand, a body that is in disharmony . . . . in this state, whatever we have grown insensible to through habit becomes sensible through the application of Magnetism. This is so because the proportion of the dissonance is increased by such application." This explains why the application of Animal Magnetism often increases the patient's *initial* discomfort. After the necessary crisis, however, the symptoms abate and the patient becomes insensitive to Animal Magnetism.

The final aphorisms in this section are worthy of note. M217-220: "The development of symptoms occurs in an inverse order to that by which the malady was formed. We might represent the disease as a ball of twine which unwinds itself in the reverse order of which it began and by which it increased. No illness can be cured without a crisis. In a crisis one should observe three stages: perturbation, coction (literally a "cooking" or coming to the boiling point) and evacuation." By "evacuation" Mesmer meant the throwing off of the poisonous material via vomiting, bowel movement, hemorrhage, sweating, etc., as well as emotional expressions well known to every medical orgone therapist.

The next section of special interest in our study is titled "Observations on Nervous Diseases." Maxim 241 states: "The exaggerated irritability of the nerves produced by the aberration of harmony within the human body, is what we designate *nervous diseases.*" Time and again Mesmer demonstrated that he could "extend the faculties" of patients with nervous disorders—in much the same manner as one uses and focuses a microscope and telescope. Such patients who underwent Animal Magnetism were enabled to see, smell, hear, and "touch" objects at great distances. *Right here is the key to much of what is now subsumed under ESP,* or extrasensory perception. "Until now, human intelligence has not dreamed of increasing the external scope of our senses by increasing the condition of sensations" (M252).

And again, in M255: "If the extension of one sense [sight] has been able to produce a considerable revolution in our knowledge, what still vaster field has again opened itself to our observation if, as I believe, the extension of the faculties of each sense, can be carried as far and even farther than lenses have carried the extension of sight."

"In nervous maladies, when in a state of crisis, irritability of the retina advances to a greater degree, *and the eye becomes capable of perceiving microscopic objects. . . .* In the most obscure darkness there is still enough light for these subjects to see by. . . . They can also determine objects through opaque bodies" (M265). Astonishing as these statements may appear, by way of proof Mesmer offers his observations of patients: "One patient whom I have treated, and several others whom I have carefully observed have furnished a number of experiences. One of them perceived the pores of the skin as of a considerable size. She described the structure in conformity with what the microscope has taught us. But she went further: The skin appeared as a sieve to her. Through it she saw the texture of the muscles, all at the correct locations, and the junction of bones in passages devoid of pulp. All this she described in an ingenious way, and was sometimes impatient at the sterility and insufficiency of our expressions for communicating ideas" (M267).

It was this same patient who described to Mesmer "all the poles of the human body clearly, as a luminous vapor— not that it was like fire, but the impression which it made upon her gave her the idea akin to fire, which she could only express by the word *light*" (M269).

Phenomena such as the following gave Mesmer much

food for thought, leading to his firm belief in the existence of his postulated Universal Fluid:

"On my face [the patient] perceived . . . luminous rays which emanated from the eyes and joined with the rays from the nose, reinforcing them. From there, they were directed toward the nearest point opposite to them. However, if I wished to observe objects to one side, without turning my head, then the rays from the eyes separated from the rays of my nose and proceeded in the direction I wished them to go. Each tip of the eyelashes, eyebrows, and hairs give a feeble light. The neck appears slightly luminous, the chest dimly lighted. If I present my hands to her, the thumb becomes immediately distinguished by a vivid light, the little finger being half as much, the index and third fingers seem lighted by only a borrowed light. The middle finger is obscure. The palm of the hand is also luminous" (M273 and 274).

The sense of sight is not the only sense thus affected: "Many times," writes Mesmer, "I have observed a person affected with nervous maladies who could not listen to the sound of a horn without falling into the strongest crisis. Frequently I have observed her complain that she heard one and finish by falling into very strong convulsions, saying that it [the sound of the horn] was approaching her. And it was only after more than a quarter of an hour later that I was able to hear it. We will observe the same phenomena for taste. Of twenty foods that we diluted to an extreme degree, a person in crisis, in whom irritability was considerably increased on the tongue and palate, could perceive a variety of tastes and flavors in these foods.

"I know a very spiritual person whose nerves are extremely irritable, who, having this irritation uniquely on the tongue, and maintaining her judgment, has told me: 'In eating this small piece of bread, as large as the head of a pin, it seems that I have a considerable mouthful, of an exquisite flavor. But what is quite singular is the fact that not only do I sense the flavor of a fine morsel of bread, but also I sense separately the taste of all the particles which compose it: the water, the farina, all finally produce upon me a multitude of sensations that I cannot express . . . which cannot be appreciated in words" (M281 and 282).

Practice of Animal Magnetism

Up to this point the skeptical reader might say, "Very interesting, but so far you have not presented any evidence to contradict the possibility that all of the patients referred to were merely *hypnotized*." There is truth to this statement. However, let me point out that although there are indeed "somnambulistic phenomena" evident in Animal Magnetism, nevertheless it is incumbent upon those who are serious students of this subject to keep several points in mind. First, at no time, as we shall now observe, did Dr. Mesmer ever use the *suggestive, inductive techniques* that are the methods of the professional and medical hypnotist. He did not *suggest* to his patients what they would or would not experience; rather, his research consisted of a definite physical method. Once his patients were affected by Animal Magnetism, their reactions, their expressions, their experiences were entirely *voluntary and unsought!* The second point to keep in mind is Mesmer's general postulation of a Universal Fluid (the biological Life Energy discovered by Dr. Wilhelm Reich). It is my firm belief that Reich's orgone energy provides Mesmer's Animal Magnetism with a firm base in physiology and biophysics. The advocates of "hypnotism" are constrained to show how the theory and practice of hypnotism can duplicate entirely the practice of Animal Magnetism, as described herein. Furthermore, from the facts given here, the proponents of hypnotism must also develop a theory consistent with all of the physical and psychological conditions, and changes of conditions, in a way that makes all such phenomena comprehensible and *leads to further development*. A theory is of no value if it gains no new insights in the field under investigation; in fact, such a theory actually obstructs further research.

The following material taken from the *Maxims* should indicate conclusively that Franz Anton Mesmer was, in truth, utilizing a physical, tangible therapeutic process that in no rational way can be considered to be "hypnotism!"

"We have seen from my Doctrine that everything in the universe is contiguous by means of a Universal Fluid in which all bodies are immersed" (M285).

Now we face the important question: *"Exactly how do we communicate the currents of the Universal Fluid to a sick individual?"*

"There are many ways to establish and strengthen [the currents of the Universal Fluid] upon man," writes Dr. Mesmer. "The surest way is to place oneself in opposition to the person one wishes to touch—that is, face to face, so that we present our right side to the left side of the patient. In order to establish harmony with him, we must place our hands upon the patient's shoulders, then proceed slowly downward along the length of the arms as far as the tips of the fingers, holding the patient's thumbs for a moment. We repeat this procedure two or three times, after which we establish the currents from the head to the feet" (M287).

The physician does not talk to his patient. He does not suggest that the patient's eyes are getting heavy, that his eyelids are drooping, that he feels sleepy. No—Mesmer is employing a *physical* therapy, *touch!* He is "communicating" his own biological energy to the patient through his hands and fingers.

"We search out the cause and site of the illness and pain," Mesmer continues. "It is, more often, by touch and reasoning that you may assure yourself of the seat and the cause of the malady and pain, which in the majority of illnesses *resides in the side opposite to the pain,* especially in paralysis, rheumatism, and other illnesses of this type" (M287).

Mesmer further describes his physical procedures as follows:

"Having fully assured yourself in this preliminary procedure, you constantly touch the cause of the malady, *maintaining the symptomatic pains, until you have rendered them critical.* In this way you assist nature's effort against the cause of the malady, and you occasion a salutary crisis, *which is the sole means of curing thoroughly.*" The physician "assuages the pains which we call 'symptomatic symptoms,' which yield to the touch, without as yet acting upon the cause of the malady." In other words, as the "symptomatic symptoms" diminish, simultaneously, or immediately thereafter, the "critical symptoms" become aggravated or irritated. Then, the critical symptoms give way to a crisis, and the patient's "malady becomes relieved, and the cause of the malady diminished" (M288).

Now let us peruse some additional, pertinent Maxims in this section:

M289: "The seat of almost all maladies is ordinarily in the viscera of the lower belly: the stomach, spleen, liver, the omentum, mesentery, kidneys, etc. The cause of all maladies or aberrations is an engorgement, obstruction, disturbance or suppression of circulation in a part which, compressing the blood vessels or lymphatics, and especially the nerve branches . . . . occasion a spasm or tension within the parts wherein they lead, especially in those parts where the fibers have less natural elasticity, as in the brain, lungs, etc., or in those parts where fluid circulates sluggishly and thickly, like the synovia, destined to facilitate movement and articulation. If these engorgements compress a nerve trunk or a considerable part of a branch, the movement and sensibility of the parts to which it corresponds are entirely suppressed, as in apoplexy, paralysis, etc."

M290: "In addition to the primary reason for touching the viscera first (that is, in order to discover the cause of the malady) there is one other determining reason: The nerves are the best conductors of Magnetism in the body. The nerves are in such great numbers within the viscera that many physicians have considered this to be the seat of the sensations of the soul. Most abundant and sensible are the nervous center of the diaphragm, the solar plexus, umbilical, etc. This mass of an infinity of nerves corresponds with all parts of the body."

M291: "One touches, in the position previously indicated, with the thumb and index finger, or with the palm of the hand, or with one finger alone reinforced by the others, by describing a line on the part that we wish to touch, and in following as closely as possible the direction of the nerves. One touches also with all five fingers open and slightly curved. Touching at a short distance from the part is stronger, because a current exists between the hand or the conductor and the patient."

M292: "One can touch indirectly with advantage by using a foreign conductor. Most commonly we use a short rod, about ten to fifteen inches long. . . . After glass, which is the best conductor, we can use iron, steel, gold, silver . . . preferring the denser material. . . . If the rod is magnetized its action is greater. However, you should permit the circumstances to determine what should be used. In the case of inflammation of the eyes, for example, or too great redness and inflammation, etc., it would be harmful. . . . In using a foreign conductor the polarity is changed, and we therefore touch differently when using a conductor—that is, from right to right and from left to left."

M293: "It is also good to oppose one pole to the other. That is, if one touches the head, the chest, the stomach, etc., with the right hand, he should oppose the left hand to the posterior part, mainly along the line separating the body in two parts, that is, from the center of the forehead to the pubis. The body represents a magnet, and once you establish the north to the right side, the left side becomes the south, and the midline the equator, which is without any predominant action. In such opposition of one hand to the other, you establish polarity."

M294: "One reinforces the action of Magnetism by multiplying the currents upon the patient. There are many more advantages to touching face to face than any other way: all the currents emanating from your viscera and from all the extensions of the body establish a circulation with the patient. The same consideration indicates the usefulness of trees, ropes, irons, chains, etc."

General Considerations of Animal Magnetism

In the previous section dealing with the actual application of Animal Magnetism, we see that Mesmer has presented us with a physical process for dealing with disease.

There is not the slightest mention or allusion to "suggestion," nor is there any indication that the patient is to be placed in a sleeping state. *Touch* is the basis of Animal Magnetism and the principal means of treatment. The fact that certain patients developed "somnambulism" was simply a phase in the therapy of those persons, especially those afflicted with what Mesmer described as "nervous irritability." Such somnambulistic states gradually disappeared and ceased to exist as the patient approached the state of health with continued treatment.

As with so many other vital discoveries, those physicians and students who practiced Animal Magnetism became enthralled by the somnambulistic phenomena, which are extremely dramatic. It was somnambulism that, distorted and divorced from Mesmer's theoretical basis in the Universal Fluid, developed into what is commonly referred to as "hypnotism." With these points in mind, let us return to Mesmer's *Maxims*.

M314: "Since it is not my intention to give a general history of illnesses and their treatment, we will cite only those which offer themselves most often to treatment by Magnetism, and the manner of applying it according to observations. . . ."

M315: "*In epilepsy,* we touch the head, on the top or at the base of the nose with one hand and the knuckles of the other. We seek the main causes, which usually converge in the viscera, and the engorgement, which in the epileptic is situated within the brain (upon which we began), and thus activate almost all the nerves of the system. *Catalepsy* is treated in the same manner."

M316: "In *apoplexy* our touching proceeds upon the main organs, such as the breast, stomach, especially the site we call 'the pit' (below the xiphoid cartilage), the site of the nervous center of the diaphragm, which reunites many nerves. We also touch, by opposition, the spinal column—tracing it to the large intercostal muscles, which are situated an inch or two from the spine, from the neck to the base of the trunk. *We must persist until we obtain crisis,* and gather all possible means of intensifying the Magnetism, either by the iron rod or a chain of human beings [who stand one behind the other, hands touching each other's shoulders—JE] which you form with as many persons as you can assemble. . . ."

M317: "In *diseases of the ear,* and in cases of deafness, as in paralysis wherein speech is impeded, and with mutes, touching is done by placing the thumbs in the ear, spreading the other fingers and presenting them to the currents of the magnetic fluid, or by gathering the currents at a distance and bringing them back with the palm of the hand to the head, where we apply the hand for some time."

M318: "*Illnesses of the eyes* are treated with the iron rod or with the end of the fingers, which we present to the part, and which we use in stroking [at a distance] the eyeball and the eyelid. We also use the rod especially in cases of *cataract.* In case of inflammation of the eyes, one should touch with extreme lightness.

M320: "*Tumors of all kinds, lymphatic and sanguine engorgements, sores,* and even *ulcers* experience excellent results. Lotions with magnetized water, local baths with such water, either cold or tepid, and the usual treatment, bring about astonishing results."

M322: "Disorders of the head are touched on the front, the

top, at the parietals, the frontal sinus, and the brow, and on the stomach and other viscera which contain the cause."

M323: "Disorders of the *teeth* are treated by touching upon the articulations of the jaws and related parts."

M325: "In *speech difficulties*, or the total negation occasioned chiefly through paralysis, we magnetize the mouth with the iron rod and the exterior of the motor muscles of this organ by touching them."

M326: "The same methods are employed in disorders of the neck, chiefly at the lymphatics. Also we magnetize the pituitary membrane, so that it likewise is joined to the other parts in treatment, and to the affects of those parts which are spread to the chest."

M327: "In *migraine headaches* we touch the stomach and temporal regions, where the pain is felt."

M328: "*Asthma*, oppression, and other affections of the chest are touched on such parts, by slowly passing the hand over the chest, and the other along the spine, allowing them to remain for a time upon the upper part, and descending slowly to the stomach, where the hand remains also."

M329: "The patient with nightmares is treated in the same manner [as asthma], instructing him not to lie upon his back until he is cured."

M330: "Pain, engorgements, obstructions of the stomach, liver, spleen and the other viscera are touched locally, and require time and perseverance. . . ."

M331: "In *colic,* vomiting, nervous irritability, and intestinal pain, as well as in pain in the lower abdomen, we touch the source of pain very lightly. In cases where inflammation exists, or inflammatory disposition, *we must avoid frictional touching of any kind.*"

M332: "In disorders of the womb, one touches not only the viscera, but also the breasts, the site of the ovaries, and the large ligaments in the lateral and posterior parts. In accordance with observations, the palm applied to the vulva expedites the menstrual flow and remedies leakages; this application is beneficial also in cases of dropping of the womb and weakening of the muscles of the vagina."

Concerning Crisis

M333: "A disease cannot be cured without a crisis. The crisis is an effort of nature against the disease, tending, through an increase of movement, tone, and intension, through the action of the magnetic fluid, to disperse the obstacles which impede circulation, and to dissolve and evacuate the obstacles which form such obstructions, thus reestablishing harmony and equilibrium within all parts of the body."

M334: "Crises can be more or less evident, more or less salutary, natural, or provoked."

M335: "Natural crises should be attributed only to the natural constitution, which acts effectively upon the cause of the malady, and which rids the body of such causes by different excretions—as in fevers, wherein the natural constitution alone overthrows that which is harmful to it, and expels it by vomiting, movement of the bowels, sweating, urinating, hemorrhagic flow, etc."

M336: "The less evident crises are those in which the natural constitution acts insensibly, without violence, by slowly breaking down the obstacles which constrict the circulation, and drives them away through insensible processes."

M337: "When the natural constitution is insufficient to establish crises, we aid it through Magnetism, which, utilized by the means indicated, in connection with the natural constitution, brings about the desired results. It is beneficial when, after experiencing a crisis, the patient feels comfortable and relieved, and chiefly when it is followed by advantageous evacuations."

M338: ". . . . When we decide that the crisis has reached its limit, which is indicated by a calm, we allow it to terminate itself. Or, when we believe it to be sufficient, we retire the patient to the state of sleep and insensibility in which he is rested."

M341: "In cases of erethism, or irritability, and of excessive susceptibility to such, it is dangerous to provoke and maintain unduly strong crises. . . . "

M342: "When we excite violent crises in one disposed to them, we maintain in the organs a condition *of forced elasticity.* . . . Such an habitual state (of forced elasticity) is detrimental to the efforts of nature. It increases the aberration and causes a wrinkle or fold to form within the organs, similar to a crease in material, which is very difficult to efface."

M343: "We observe on the one hand the advantage and necessity of crises; and on the other hand the misuse which we can make of them."

M344: "A physician who is schooled in the doctrine of Animal Magnetism and who is an accurate observer of the effects of crises will be able to derive from them all the benefits which they afford and will guard himself against the dangers of their abuse."

Wherefore I put thee in remembrance that thou stir up
the gift of God, which is in thee by the putting on of my
hands.

(2 Timothy 1:6)

3 Case Histories

We now turn our attention to the application of Animal Magnetism to sick people. Most of these cases were first brought to public attention through the pages of *The Zoist*, edited and published by Dr. John Elliotson and his associates more than a century ago, despite a growing storm of scathing contempt and ridicule by their scientific contemporaries.

Let us approach these cases with an open mind and a positive attitude, both of which are indispensable in true scientific inquiry where basically *new* phenomena are to be scrutinized. In various passages we shall meet with language that, because of its age, presents us with some minor linguistic problems. Wherever possible, I have chosen to present the original words and phrases employed. Minor material, as well as extraneous matter, has been cut and edited.

Case 1: Epilepsy

Mr. Chenevix found an opportunity to renew his trials of mesmerism with a woman, age 34, who had labored for six years under severe epilepsy and had lately in a fit fallen into a fire and "most dreadfully burnt her leg." She also had a strong tendency to paralysis of the left leg and thigh, and was subject to almost daily spasmodic contractions of the hands and feet, accompanied by wracking pain, which sometimes lasted twelve hours or more. The woman had occasional lapses of mind and loss of memory, never slept more than a few hours at a time. She was constantly thirsty and her appetite was bad. She was eight months advanced in her sixth pregnancy, and it was after her first confinement that she had her first attack.

1st Day: Mr. Chenevix mesmerized her for forty-five minutes and produced only a little drowsiness, but that night she slept better than usual and had no spasms.

2nd Day: Mesmerized her for forty-five minutes, but no sleep, only drowsiness.

3rd Day: Mesmerized her forty-five minutes, but no sleep.

4th Day: Not mesmerized.

5th Day: Fell asleep after being mesmerized for nine minutes. She felt stronger and better than before the treatment was begun. The spasms had returned but lasted a shorter time than usual.

6th Day: Not mesmerized, and she had no spasms except in one foot for a few minutes.

7th Day: She went to sleep after three minutes; but she awoke on being spoken to. Now all this in an ignorant peasant was so beautifully conformable to the daily experience of mesmerizers. Had she been faking, she would not have awakened as soon as spoken to and her health would not have improved.

8th Day: Mesmerized.

9th Day: Not mesmerized.

10th and 11th Days: Fell into complete mesmeric sleep in two minutes. Her health was improving rapidly.

12th and 13th Days: Not mesmerized.

14th Day: Put to sleep in six minutes *by will alone,* without any visible manifestation.

[*Note:* The presence of the Magnetizer was in itself "ample manifestation," inasmuch as his biological energy field was operating upon and interacting with the energy field of the patient. JE]

15th Day: Not mesmerized.

16th Day: The woman was mesmerized *through the door at a distance of fifteen feet*—she not knowing that she was being acted upon, but supposing that I was absent. In fourteen minutes she was in complete mesmeric sleep. [Note: Mesmer mentions how various patients may be affected at a distance with Animal Magnetism—just as a compass needle may be affected by fluctuations in the magnetic field surrounding it. This phenomenon occurs many times in the literature, particularly in those patients suffering from "nervous irritability." Apparently, epilepsy falls in this category.]

17th Day: Not mesmerized, and during this interval of two days without mesmerism she had a severe attack of spasms in her left thigh and leg for six hours, followed by coldness and numbness.

18th Day: Asleep in half a minute. Her left limbs were thereupon mesmerized for forty minutes, and then she was awakened, when the pain was absolutely gone and her limbs had recovered their usual strength and heat. This was the last return of these symptoms, for by this time she had completely recovered her ability to sleep, not only at night, but was frequently obliged to lie down in the day. She now slept ten or twelve hours in the twenty-four, and one day for sixteen hours. She continued rapidly to improve her health, and her appearance was so much changed that her neighbors, who knew nothing of her treatments, were struck at the alteration. Mesmerism was continued until June 20th, when her pregnancy made her unable to come out, and on June 28th she was delivered.

On July 6th, Mr. Chenevix called upon her and found her

up and well, except for rheumatic pains in her left shoulder, for which he mesmerized her. She soon felt the pains *descending to her elbow* and thence to her wrist, and in less than ten minutes she was perfectly relieved.

July 17: She went to thank Mr. Chenevix for her recovery. *And neither then nor afterwards was he able to affect her again with mesmerism.* [After a successful treatment, the inability to affect the patient further with Animal Magnetism was considered by Mesmer to be the criterion of cure.]

Mr. Chenevix sums up this interesting case:

Nine months after the cessation of treatment, her fits had not returned. From the very first day that she was mesmerized the symptoms were alleviated and decreased regularly as the treatment advanced. In less than a week, thirst, sleeplessness, shivering, and pains *to which she had been subject for six years ceased!* The paralytic tendency diminished, and the spasmodic contractions were entirely removed after the twelfth day of mesmerizing.

Although none of the extraordinary symptoms of lucidity occurred, and although this patient awoke the instant she was spoken to, her cure is interesting as being completed so rapidly. Twenty-one sittings sufficed. Even during the period when she was most affected by mesmerism, the touch of my finger, so slight as to be almost imperceptible to myself, roused her from her state of mesmerism with the sensation which she described as "like the prick of a pin." I have known some educated persons who have experienced a similar sensation, comparing it to "an electric spark."

Case 2: Consumption

Dr. Cotter had for some time attended a poor man named Michael Donelly and pronounced him "far advanced in rapid consumption." Mr. Chenevix found the man in bed, exceedingly weak, his voice scarcely audible. He was taking small but repeated doses of tartar emetic and digitalis.

All medications were stopped, and Mr. Chenevix mesmerized him for the first time on February 11. The only sensible affect at the time was profuse perspiration. The patient thereupon slept for about an hour, and upon awakening found his cough and breathing easier.

Feb. 12: He was mesmerized again with the same results.

Feb. 13: His voice was stronger and he seemed more alive than Mr. Chenevix had yet seen him. Mr. Chenevix left him to be mesmerized by his wife for thirty minutes, night and morning. [Note: the application of Animal Magnetism is quite arduous, and it was not uncommon for the attending physician to use others, especially those of the same household, to apply Magnetism as prescribed.]

Feb. 27: Mr. Chenevix called and found the patient up and dressed. He received Mr. Chenevix at the door of his cottage, spoke with a strong, firm voice, looked healthy, and said he was nearly recovered.

March 16: The patient went to see Mr. Chenevix and looked quite well. Mr. Chenevix mesmerized him for a few minutes. He slept and showed some interesting phenomena. Mr. Chenevix urged the wife to continue the treatments for some time longer, as Animal Magnetism, when persevered in after the cure is affected is never dangerous.

This case, Mr. Chenevix adds, can be attested by at least twenty witnesses of the first respectability. When he informed Dr. Cotter that he had undertaken this desperate case, that physician's reply was: "If the poor man is saved, I will substitute the pronoun 'you' for 'we'."

Case 3: Insanity

The clinical investigation and diagnosis of emotional disorders in the 1840s were in their infancy, as we shall see. All types of behavioral and emotional aberrations were lumped under the single heading "insanity," a word whose root meaning is simply "not healthy," which is certainly correct. Usually, "insane" persons were brought to the attention of a family physician, or were hospitalized, when gross behavior disorders made it mandatory. The modern student of human ills should find the usual course of therapy prescribed for insane people very interesting. Bleeding, blistering agents, laxatives, the massive use of drugs, and physical restraint were commonly employed. The use of Animal Magnetism on such patients provided—in contrast to the usual therapeutic procedures—a new and efficacious means of restoring formerly "hopeless" patients to health.

The first case was under the care of Dr. Wilson in Middlesex Hospital. It was in June 1838 that I [Dr. John Elliotson] witnessed the case. William Rumsey, age 31, labored under extreme depressive spirits, which rendered him unable to sleep. He walked the room all night in distraction. He could do no work nor could he apply himself in the slightest way to anything. His despondency led him frequently to contemplate suicide. He occasionally had headaches and giddiness and, at length, he hesitated in his speech.

During the last three years he had a pain in his right side, extending to his loins, which was believed to be connected with a liver complaint. He had been no less than twenty months altogether at various times during that period on the sick list.

Dr. Wilson resolved to treat the patient with mesmerism, and very striking, sensible effects were produced. The man always remained wide awake, not being even sleepy. Such phenomena took place, nevertheless, as one continually observes in those patients who are in mesmeric "sleep-waking."

After longitudinal passes with the hands were made before the patient for three or four minutes, he began to tremble all over and to have twitching. His arms and legs, and even his fingers, extended and became more or less rigid as if—in his own words—he was "being influenced by someone lightly and gently touching the ends of my fingers and drawing them apart."

All resistance to these changes he found fruitless. His arms extended backwards as far as the chair would allow. The force of extension he felt to increase and decrease as the operator's hands approached or receded from him. By movement of the operator's hands as if to draw him by attractive passes without contact, he was drawn immediately from one side to the other, forwards or backwards, as he sat with his arms and legs rigidly extended. Or his arms and hands could be drawn firmly together or separated, or made to clasp his knees, notwithstanding his every effort to resist the influence.

Dr. Wilson could produce these effects at a distance of fourteen feet. In spite of himself, the patient turned toward the mesmerizer, wherever the latter might place himself, so as to be turned on his hips in the chair, and be brought sometimes nearly off the chair, nothwithstanding great struggle to retain his proper position.

[*Note:* These phenomena of "attraction" to the mesmerizer reestablished Mesmer's belief that the human body was analogous to the magnet. It is well known that in order to magnetize a piece of iron, it is sufficient to stroke the iron against a magnet.]

If Dr. Wilson went into the next room, so that merely the points of his fingers could be seen, the influence still ensued.

In performing tractive passes, the effects were greater the nearer the operator's hands were to the patient. So great was the force of traction that the patient could actually be drawn off his chair onto the floor, while his arms and legs were rigid and extended. His susceptibility so increased that Dr.

Wilson could at last affect him at a distance of 112 feet. Here are the patient's own words at this point:

"When I was asked to go the distance of 112 feet from the operator, I laughed at the idea, thinking it impossible to be affected at this great distance. In less than five minutes, however, I was so much affected as to cause me to extend my arms, and my legs would likewise have extended had I not been in a standing position, supported at the back by a wall. During the time that Dr. Wilson was acting upon me at this great distance, a friend of his that was present stepped between us at a distance of about six feet from me. His doing so appeared to deter the power of the magnetism for a few seconds, but when standing there for a few seconds it appeared to return with its full strength, so much so that I was compelled to request the doctor to cease."

The patient would sometimes endeavor to think of anything else rather than the operation of Animal Magnetism, but the effects came just as certainly. He said that during the mesmerisation, *he always felt as if attached to Dr. Wilson by something flexible.*

One day I [Dr. Elliotson] attempted to influence the patient when he was under the influence of Dr. Wilson, but with no result. Dr. Wilson then placed the tips of his fingers near the back of the patient's hands and the latter felt "as if a stream of warm water came upon them from each of Dr. Wilson's fingers and flowed to the end of my own fingers." And Dr. Wilson's power seemed greater than it had ever been before. The man's lips could be moved and his mouth drawn open by tractive passes before them with the fingers—an experiment I often made with my patient Elizabeth Okey.

After being mesmerised, the patient was always weak, tremulous, and gapish for a short time, though not at all sleepy. But this wore off in about two hours, and he slept soundly at night. The very first night, after having been mesmerised in the day, he slept much better, and the pain in his right side and back (which no doubt was the neuralgic pain like those of the right or left side in so many young females and called, as it generally is in them, a proof of liver disease) was lessened. After the second session with mesmerism he slept soundly all night and was much better.

After having been mesmerised thirteen times he was perfectly well. His first treatment was begun on June 15, and the patient was discharged as cured on August 2, and went to his occupation.

Case 4: Melancholia

This is the case of a very robust, healthy-looking mother, 30 years of age, Mrs. S. She had suffered two or three attacks of nervousness, but in the summer of 1841 fell into a state of absolute distraction. She fancied all sorts of misfortunes, and like so many melancholy patients, now that mesmerism is a subject of general conversation, adopted the delusion of having suffered from mesmerism. She imagined that a discharged maidservant had "mesmerised her," and that a child which she had lost was "not dead, but had been mesmerised away from her." She told me [Dr. Elliotson] that "you know all this very well."

The woman would cry bitterly, wring her hands and grow frantic, accuse all her friends of injuring her, fall into the most furious rage, and talk incessantly of her imagined afflictions. She wished to destroy herself, begged others to kill her, and yet was distractedly anguished with the conviction that she would die and never recover.

All attempts of persuasion were lost upon her. She complained of a scalding pain inside her head and down her arms, and in the paroxysms of despair and rage—for she was worse at times every day and night—her face was flushed. She hardly ever slept. Her bowels required laxatives every day, but her tongue was clean and moist, and her pulse was about 90, and not at all full. She had lived sparingly, but I allowed her to eat meat and she frequently ate well. Sometimes she refused both food and the laxative, being resolved "never to swallow anything again."

The only medicine calculated to tranquillize her distracted feelings was opium. And finding, from her medical attendant, that he had given her one-half grain of morphine with no effect, I ordered her one grain immediately and another at bedtime, if she did not sleep. This was May 18, 1841. She became calmer and less fearful with the morphine, but did not sleep; however, she was soon as bad as ever, and it was necessary to increase the dose and frequency of the morphine. Finally, we had to augment the dose to four and one-half drams once or even twice a day before sleep was produced, and then to increase this dose to five and six drams.

Finally, it was decided that no further opiates should be given, and Mr. Wood began mesmerising her for me on September 11. Following are the notes of Mr. Wood:

The patient was mesmerised the first time for fifteen minutes, whereupon she fell asleep. Continued mesmerising her for half an hour and then left her asleep. *The patient slept ten hours and is evidently better but will not acknowledge it.* I continued mesmerising her, at regular intervals. While awake, the patient constantly complains and moans: "It's of no use; it's of no use. I am sure nothing will do me any good." Mesmerised her and procured sleep in about the same time as yesterday, and left her asleep.

September 13: The patient slept twelve hours from the time I left her, and then she awoke in what they called a choking fit and was very sick. The sickness continued and a medical attendant was sent for, and he gave her a dose of morphine. She appeared to be under the influence of it when I saw her, but the sickness continued. I did not mesmerise her, as the morphine had so unfortunately been given her by the medical attendant.

September 14: She had no sleep last night. Mesmerised her as usual. After twenty minutes she fell asleep and I left her asleep. [Note: One can only conjecture about the efficacy of Animal Magnetism in cases of drug addiction. JE]

September 15: She only slept for two hours. Sickness continues. Sent her to sleep as usual.

September 16: Sleep did not continue after I left her. Sickness is better.

September 17: Rather better. More quiet, though she had very little sleep last night. Here the mischief of giving morphine was evident—*it prevented the full effects of mesmerism for days.*

September 20: Improving, but does not sleep much except while being mesmerised. When mesmerised her sleep is sometimes very profound and she snores, but it does not continue after I leave her.

September 25: She will not acknowledge that she is any better, but she certainly is very much better. Appetite greatly improved and strength increased. She is able to walk across the room. The improvement is obvious to everyone but herself.

September 29: She is getting stronger every day. Always sleeps when mesmerised, but very little any other time. She takes no aperient (laxative) medicine.

October 5: Getting stronger daily. She sleeps better but still not soundly. The improvement continues daily.

October 21: Is now able to sit up and is steadily improving.

November 10: Able to come down stairs. Sleeps better. Still has a good deal of headache.

November 25: She has actually gone out of the house, and seems all the better for it!

December 3: There is still occasionally some headache, but in other respects she is pretty well, though rather weak.

December 26: She spent the day yesterday away from home, and is none the worse.

December 30: She continues very well. The lady remains well to this hour—nearly two years having elapsed.

Case 5: Insanity

The following case is presented by Dr. Elliotson. Again we see the salutary effect of Animal Magnetism as a *physical* therapy, utilizing only the hands of the physician, without verbal, suggestive techniques of any kind.

The case involves Master Linnell of Mercer Road, Northampton. The boy, nine years of age, was characterized as "a clever and healthy lad and always in action." While reading by the fire, on Friday, November 4, 1842, the boy was suddenly frightened by flames descending from the chimney. The communicating chimney of the kitchen below had caught fire. The boy screamed and ran out of the room. That night, after he had been in bed for two hours, he flew screaming downstairs, as white as a sheet, saying that he smelled fire, and that the fire had broken out again. His mother warmed him, gave him some wine, and put him to bed again. In another hour he ran down screaming again in fright. His mother then kept him with her until she went to bed herself.

On Saturday he was poorly, fretting and low in spirits. On Sunday at church he disturbed his mother by fidgetiness during the whole of the service, on which account she punished him. On Monday and Tuesday he was observed to be in great agitation, and his mouth frothed, which he said he could not help, for his "tongue was grown so large." He spoke so badly that his mother thought he was mimicking and scolded him. He cried and said he could not speak properly. She saw that he was ill and supposed the fright had been the cause. A druggist told her that the fright "had caused too much blood to flow to the brain and that he might have worms," but that by giving a little medicine and plenty of nourishment he would soon get better. The druggist sent him three powders.

In a statement which she drew up, the mother writes: "I gave him two of the powders, and after the action on the bowels he was immediately worse. But finding him get worse, I sent him to Dr. Robertson who said it was the St. Vitus' Dance, caused by fright, and ordered him a blister on the back of the neck and strengthening medicines. The next day I was obliged to send for Dr. Robertson, as the motions had increased so much that he could not hold himself and he had quite lost his speech. Dr. Robertson and Mr. Terry, a surgeon, attended him daily for some time, and he had scarcely any sleep for ten nights, and took a great deal of medicine and a shower bath every morning.

"Not seeing him get better I asked the doctor if a change might not be of use. He said certainly. I brought him to London and, having read a book of the Reverend W. W. Mosely, took my child to him. But after a week's trial found him getting worse and was obliged to hire a carriage to draw him in and out of the house. I then went to Surgeon Chumley of Nottingham Place, who said he seldom saw a case of that kind cured in boys."

The mother was advised by Mr. Dyer of upper Marylebone Street to bring him to me [Dr. John Elliotson].

On January 4, 1843, the boy was brought in a coach to

me and obliged to be carried into the house. Supported by his mother he walked with great difficulty from my dining room into my library. His debility was such that he could not stand a moment unsupported. His head hung on one side, his tongue out of his mouth, which constantly slobbered. His look was quite fatuitous.

He could not articulate, making only inarticulate noises, and these with extreme difficulty. Even "yes" and "no" were said in the strangest manner, so as hardly to be understood. He often fell into a passion, not being able to articulate. He ground his teeth and sighed greatly, continually blew bubbles of saliva from his mouth, and moved his tongue. He could use neither hand for any purpose, and scarcely ever raised the right. He was low-spirited and fretful, and often cried. His tongue was clear and moist, his appetite good, and his bowels in the most healthy condition. Pulse, 74.

He cried sadly at being brought to me, thinking that I should give him loads of physics to swallow, and blister him as others had done. I mesmerised him by vertical passes before his face for half an hour. He sat well supported in an easy chair, his hand on his breast. But he sat so quietly in comparison with his usual state that his mother noticed it. He was mesmerised daily for the same time in the same way.

January 5, 6: Spoke less inarticulately after mesmerism today than before. He can walk and stand alone a little.

January 7: Walks with less support. His countenance is clearer and its expression more intelligent. Perfectly still while mesmerised. Walks better after being mesmerised. Walked twice around the room alone, without stopping, though unsteadily, and he stood well alone.

January 9: Walked alone four times around the room after being mesmerised. Is always much stronger after it than before.

January 10, 11: Walked five times alone around the room and without stopping, faster and much upright.

January 12, 13: Walks much better and speaks better. Said, "Pudding." He blows no bubbles with his saliva while mesmerised, and has gaped as if sleepy for several days during the process.

January 14, 15: Walks still better and speaks decidedly better.

January 17: Stands about the room well and has walked out of doors alone twice. Articulates a great many words. He has sat less and less drooping and supported while being mesmerised. Has sighed, slobbered, and blown bubbles less and less. In a few days he read aloud freely in a book opened by me at random, and took a walk every day. In three weeks from the first day of mesmerism, he fed himself with his left hand and walked from his lodgings in Park Street, Dorse Square, to my house.

January 30: He walked five miles and could talk well. He continued to improve rapidly. He could use his right hand well on the 2nd of February.

By February 10th he was perfectly cured. At this time (June 26) he continues perfectly well.

Case 6: Epilepsy

This treatment of an epileptic child was reported by Dr. John Elliotson. Interestingly enough, Dr. Elliotson undertook the case at the time he was ordered to cease his practice of Animal Magnetism or leave his post at University Hospital. The doctor left the hospital.

Master Salmon, the son of Mr. Salmon, an old established and most respectable mercer* of 22 Red Lion Street,

---

*A mercer is one who dealt in textiles.

Holborn, was born in April 1826. In 1834, when he was eight years of age, he began to have attacks of violent pains in the abdomen, and, if in a carriage at the time, he would vomit. Dr. Roots, Dr. Conquest, Dr. Pierce, and all the other medical men who were consulted were understood to say that the glands of the abdomen were too large, so that the pain was evidently ascribed to "mesenteric disease."

I have no doubt it was neuralgia, as epileptics, hysterics, and other persons laboring under nervous diseases are very liable to neuralgic pains—sometimes agonizing—before, during, and after the epileptic or hysterical attacks, and chiefly in the head and abdomen. And in the latter situation, mesenteric, hepatic, or other visceral affections are generally declared to exist.

That the boy had no mesenteric disease is certain, for he never has had any sign of such affection: no enlargement, no emaciation, et cetera—nothing but the attack of pain for a time. An abdominal pain is not alone sufficient ground for the hypothetical opinion of the existence of hepatic or mesenteric affection. But medical men every day give groundless opinions.

In 1836, while suffering from a severe attack of this kind, he was seized with an universal shaking and stiffness which lasted twenty minutes. A similar seizure, in all respects, took place the next morning, and a third in the evening. His head was drawn back at the time. The attacks came about three times a day for three months, then more and more frequently and severely, always morning and evening, and soon after meals. After these attacks had recurred for a year, perfect epilepsy took place.

In the epileptic fits he was perfectly insensible, bit his tongue, foamed, he required many persons to hold him, and once tore away from four men. The usual duration of these attacks was one hour. He was again attended a fortnight by

Dr. Roots, who purged him strongly with calomel and other things, but he got worse than ever and began to bark loudly during the whole attack. He had no warning, but would be seized while speaking to or kissing his mother, and remained in a comatose state for an hour or two after the fit. There was but one continued fit—not a succession united as in hysteria. And he had about one every day, but at one time only on a Sunday. I have in a few cases noticed the recurrence to take place on particular days for a time, and frequently on a Sunday.

After leaving Dr. Roots, he was placed under Dr. Lane for a year and a half, but with no success. All sorts of remedies were tried in vain. After a fit, an arm or a leg would occasionally remain paralyzed for a short time. In other cases I have seen impaired motion or insensibility of some part or other after a fit, and sometimes violent neuralgic pain and tenderness of a part, accordingly as portions of the nervous system devoted to sensation or motion happened to be affected, and according to the way in which they were affected.

He had suffered neuralgia before the epilepsy and was now subject to palsy after the attacks. Once his lower extremities remained palsied for a fortnight so that he could not stand; and then another fit took place and perfectly restored them. He once lost the use of his side for two days, and once his speech for half a day.

On January 26, 1839, I was summoned to him late in the afternoon and found him lying on a couch so paralyzed that not only could he not walk, but he could not raise his head in the least from the pillow, or move his head to one side. If others raised him even a few inches, he became insensible, or, as the family said, "fainted." Of all this I satisfied myself.

A fit which had taken place twelve days before had left

him thus paralyzed in the legs and trunk and neck. Though I had just resigned at University College, because I was not allowed to cure my patients with mesmerism, the boy's father had no opinion on mesmerism and gave me ink, pen, and paper to write a prescription. But knowing, as all medical men in their hearts do, that medicine in the majority of cases of epilepsy and numerous other nervous affections is of no or little or of secondary use—whatever number of pills in bottles are consumed—I said nothing, but went to my carriage and requested Mr. Wood, who was in it, to come and help me mesmerise a patient. We returned to the house.

I raised the child to the sitting posture, and almost immediately he became comatose, as many epileptic and hysterical patients are in the habit of becoming between the perfect fits, or when the perfect fits have not yet shown themselves. He was not pale, nor was his pulse altered. The state was coma, not fainting.

I restored him to the horizontal position and made transverse passes before his chest and face, and he awoke suddenly and perfectly, with the usual sudden inspiration which I had always seen characterise the Okeys* and many other mesmerised patients to the waking state. The parents said that the return to consciousness was much more rapid than they had ever seen it before, showing that his state was really mesmeric.

I then, *without a word*, took Mr. Wood's hand, and he took the father's, and with the other hand I made passes before the child's face downwards as he lay. His eyelids presently began to droop and in about five minutes they nearly closed and were in a state of rapid tremor. His jaw

---

*The Okeys were two sisters who were treated by Dr. Elliotson, and who displayed remarkable phenomena in the mesmeric state.

had become locked, and he could not be roused by rough
shaking, nor did he appear to hear, except that clapping
the hands in his face increased the tremulous contractions
of his eyelids.

I made passes along his arm and hand, and that extremity
extended and rose and presently fell. Then I made passes
transversely and the arm and hand moved transversely. On
repeating the longitudinal passes, his extremity extended
and rose again.

The child was ignorant of mesmerism and "sleep-waking"
or somnambulism, but beautifully displayed, though un-
prepared for my mesmeric proceedings, the phenomena of
mesmerism and sleep-waking. He was fast asleep, as his
breathing and indifference showed. He fell asleep in the
true mesmeric manner—his eyelids closed and trembled and
his jaw was locked.

During the whole of my attendance his eyes were always
open a little, as everybody clearly saw, and he directed them
to his mesmeriser. And when he was able—as he was in a
few days—he directed his head likewise, in order to watch
his mesmeriser. There was no disguise. He had a strong
propensity to imitate and obey and use his external senses
naturally for information. I have had patients who learnt
what was happening without any known means, and imitated
grimaces made behind them when their eyes were closed.
Persons ignorant of the subject pronounced patients like
this boy to be impostors. I did so myself in two or three
instances, when I first attended to mesmerism, and deeply
do I now lament the injustice I did to the individuals.

I was not aware that the propensity to obey and imitate
might be excited in sleep-waking, while no means beyond
the external senses existed to supply the patient with information. And when I deceived a patient and led him to
imitate what he fancied me to do, and not what I really did,

I accused him of imposition. My conscience is never easy when I think of my injustice. A young woman, in whom this was remarkably the case, angered me greatly and I scolded her and did not take any further interest in her and ceased to mesmerise her. She died of her disease in the hospital after I left town one autumn. My moments are to this day embittered when my injustice towards her recurs in my memory. My only excuse is my ignorance. I must be thankful that I did not—like my brethren—remain ignorant, but that, seeing that there was truth in mesmerism, applied myself to it til I became familiarized with its facts.

I next moved Master Salmon's legs by vertical tractive passes, and then made passes toward his head. He responded to these tractive passes by beginning to move his head with some effort. Mr. Wood and myself now made the tractive passes together, and the boy's effort became greater and greater til at last he raised his head from the pillow—a *thing he had not done for ten days*. It soon fell back again, but we persevered again and again til he rose in the sitting posture. The more we slowly retreated in making these tractive movements, the stronger appeared to be the influence. At last, after having drawn him into the sitting posture, we made tractive passes from the top of his head upwards, and this soon made him elevate his head, and then his whole frame, til he positively stood erect on the floor!

I walked backward, making tractive passes from him to me and he slowly followed me. His father and mother were petrified and called in their people from the shop to witness the strange sight of their child, with his head nodding in sleep, slowly moving after me—*unable to move his head an inch or raise his legs at all a quarter of an hour before!* The room was behind the shop and small. I opened the door, receded into the shop, and he slowly followed me.

I returned him to the room again, making the tractive passes, and he went round the room after me. I stood on one leg; he stood on one leg. I turned round; he turned round. I opened my mouth; he opened his mouth. I drew him onwards to the couch and laid him down upon it. I awoke him two or three times by blowing in his face, and sent him to sleep again presently by longitudinal passes before him.

January 27: On visiting him in the middle of the next day, he immediately raised himself on the sofa and held out his hand to me. He had experienced no headache since the preceding evening, though before he had long suffered from it.

I begged his father to drive him to my house. When he arrived, they put him in a sitting posture in an easy chair, and it was not til the end of five minutes that the insensibility took place and his hands became cold. His mother stated to the company that previously he instantly became insensible if even his head was raised enough for his nightcap to be put on. I laid him down and he soon recovered with the usual sudden inspiration. I made longitudinal passes before his face and his eyelids began to tremble and in a few minutes he was asleep.

I drew his arms and legs in different positions and directions by tractive passes and then, by means of them, drew him forward in the chair and then upwards, and he stood upright on the floor, followed me all about the room, and imitated every movement which I made.

At last I made outward passes with my thumbs on my own eyebrows. He did the same on his own, and immediately awoke to his natural state. He was in perfect ignorance of all that had happened and declared himself not in the least tired. Before he awoke, finding him quite deaf, I pointed my fingers just into his ears, and after a short period he heard. To my question whether he was asleep, he replied, "Yes." And to my second question—When would he wake if nothing were done to him? he replied, "Never."

January 28: He was now able to sit up a long while without insensibility coming on. I sent him to sleep and, standing at his right hand, drew up his legs by tractive passes. After they had dropped, I attempted to draw up his right arm in the same way, but instead, the legs came up again. I then tried the left arm. It did not rise on account of it being wedged in between the body and the side of the couch—but his right arm and both legs came up. I disengaged his left arm and, standing on his left side, endeavored to draw up his left arm, but both arms and both legs rose and continued to rise, though I ceased to make any tractive movement.

This is very curious and similar to what I continually observed. When a muscular effect has been produced—elevation, depression, or extension—*it has a strong tendency to recur* when any attempt to produce a muscular effect is made. The idea seems fixed in the patient and confounds itself with the new impression, or even gets the upper hand of it, at least for a time. Not only will the previous movement of the same sitting then return, but a movement of a former sitting.

I had a patient who, like many others, though fast asleep mesmerically, and *with his eyes bandaged,* could close or extend his hand exactly as I closed or extended mine near his—though how he knew what I did is a perfect mystery. The effect came slowly, and if I placed my fingers and thumbs in strange positions he repeated them very slowly and not til many efforts and mistakes, though at last most accurately. I had one day put my thumb between the fore and middle fingers and he had done the same. The following day I put my hand in some other position, and before he imitated this—which he at length did—he put his thumb precisely in the condition of the previous day; and for some time he continued to show a tendency to do this when I presented to his hand my closed or extended hand for him to imitate.

January 30: The boy is so strong that he sits up without any support or cushion or backrest, and walks across the room without assistance. When he was sent to sleep the attraction to me was so powerful that he not only followed me about the room but stood as close as possible to me. And when I sat down, he sat down in the same chair, pushing violently at me as if he wished to be in the very same point in space.*

The child now attempted to drive against me while standing, but soon gave up and yielded to his propensity to imitate all I did. I took a spoon off the sideboard and laid it on the floor. He did not go through the whole of this procedure but only of the latter part. He stooped down and put his hand on the floor. When I spoke, he spoke in a whisper, repeating my very words. He tried to whistle when I whistled. In following me about, he reeled so far to one side that all thought continually that it was impossible for him not to fall—yet he always righted himself and never fell.

January 31: Sleep took place with passes made at the distance of ten feet, though not so quickly as usual. I laid him flat on his back and, by tractive passes, made him rise and stand up without assistance from touching the floor with his hands. This he desired to do after he awoke, but was unable.

February 1: His health is very much improved and he

---

*This phenomenon calls to mind Wilhelm Reich's discovery of attraction and superimposition of two orgone energy units. See his book *Cosmic Superimposition.*

walks about when awake very well. Hitherto he has been mesmerised daily, but henceforth will be mesmerised only every other day.

February 2: He had a fit this morning which lasted half an hour, instead of an hour as formerly, differently from what had happened before. He both was not unconscious during the fit and was afterwards conscious of having had it. He could not think what was the matter with him while he was kicking about, and called upon his family to hold him still.

Such was *the insensibility to pain in his mesmeric sleep,* that although he had for a long time an eruption with open sores upon his head, he could bear the touching of the sores after he had been sent to sleep. His mother, noticing this insensibility, proposed sending him to sleep every day when she was going to dress the sores, as the agony he suffered was extreme. This was done ever afterwards til the head was healed. When about to dress the sores, his mother made a few passes before his face, sent him to sleep, dressed the wounds without his noticing what she did, and blew in his face and awoke him again.

February 6: Not only does his health improve, but the sores on his head have healed so much that he can bear his head touched in his waking state.

February 15: For twenty minutes he had the shaking, which is the premonitory symptom of a fit—but no fit occurred! The peevishness, which has existed during the whole of his illness, is undiminished. The treatment has consisted simply in sending him to sleep by a few passes, or pointing the fingers before his eyes and then drawing up his arms and legs, and drawing him by passes after me about the room, and talking to him.

A few medical men witnessed the case, but they merely thought it very odd and went about their business again like men wise in their generation, not pondering on such wonders and the working of the brain, nor thinking of any improvement in the confused and unsatisfactory and often absurd and injurious treatment which has been followed from generation to generation in such diseases.

A friend of mine heard a provincial surgeon, who makes four thousand pounds a year say, after witnessing a mesmeric case: "It was very funny and I never thought of it again."

March 7: In his sleep, I asked the boy if he could tell me whether he should be cured. He answered, "Yes," saying that he should have no more fits, but that he should have five indications, and those all in three months.* By "indications" he meant shakings without unconsciousness—that is, premonitory symptoms of his fits, but not followed by fits. Many epileptic persons, besides their perfect fits, have fragments of fits, abortive fits, sudden shaking, catching, or starting, or powerlessness of their limbs without consciousness, or giddiness amounting to, perhaps, momentary unconsciousness. On asking him how often I ought to mesmerise him, he left this to my judgement.

March 9: Instead of pointing to both eyes, I pointed my forefinger to one only, the right, and it alone closed. Speaking to him, he said he was not asleep but seemed rather oppressed and flushed, as he always was in his sleep. I then pointed my finger to the other eye and it instantly closed and he was asleep. He assured me again that he shall have no more fits, but five "indications" and those in the course of three months. He adds, however, that this result will depend upon my mesmerising him every day.

---

*The ability to "see" into their own physical bodies and accurately predict the course of therapy and the outcome are phenomena not uncommon in those undergoing mesmerism. Edgar Cayce, "the sleeping doctor," had this ability to an amazing degree.

On another occasion when I mesmerised one eye only, he said he was "cut in half"—that is, one half only was powerless, as in sleep.

March 18: His mother informs me that all his life he has incessantly required aperient medicines, but that since I began to mesmerise him his bowels have become more and more regular and he now never requires any. This morning, when up, he fancied he heard a number of people talking, and he was worried at it. Any noise gave him this idea. When in mesmeric sleep he tells me the same thing and remarks that being sent to sleep now seems to excite him a great deal.

I have noticed in other cases that as recovery advanced mesmerism began to excite and required to be performed less frequently. It is a fact similar to that of patients who bore and required a certain amount of food or wine or tonic medicine in the height of illness, becoming over-excited by the same quantity as they improve, and requiring gradual diminution. I judged it right, therefore, to mesmerise him but three times a week.

March 24: Has gradually stood and walked more firmly so that he never totters in his sleep-waking. Is not sent to sleep quite so easily, and certainly is not wakened without much more blowing than formerly. In his sleep-waking state, moments of deep sleep come on more frequently than before. He has often a pain or sense of weakness in his right knee, which in his sleep-waking state he says is a nervous affection.

April 3: Sleep induced certainly more slowly. The moments of deep sleep are still more frequent. And after waking, his eyes, which lately remained closed for a short time, are now more slowly brought to open by breathing or passes upon them.

April 19: He says in sleep-waking that he shall have an "indication" about once a fortnight, til they are completed.

The moments of deep sleep are more frequent. The traction movements are still easy. In his waking state his family have noticed a strong attachment to me, and he has prevailed on his father to purchase my lithographed portrait.

His predictions were fulfilled accurately. He had his five "indications," the last on the 15th of March, and he has never experienced another, nor a fit, though (at this writing) *above four years have elapsed.*

Mr. Wood and I mesmerised him every other day til midsummer, and after he was well he invariably refused to be mesmerised, being conscious of the influence over him. Last year he was troubled with headache, and a friend and myself *tried fifteen times to mesmerise him for it, but never produced the slightest effect.* He is in perfect health.

The liberal manner in which the father allowed any friend to see the phenomena, and the independent, honest manner in which the father asserted the truth of mesmerism from the first to anybody, are beyond all praise. The palsy would probably have ceased, sooner or later, spontaneously, but the instantaneous affect of mesmerism upon it was astounding. And the rapid and perfect cure of the epilepsy, without any other means, after literally "pailfulls of medicine" (to use the father's own words) had been taken in vain, was astounding.

The cure of the sore head and the establishment of healthy action in the bowels, after years of caustiveness, were very striking.

Case 7: Deafness and Dumbness

This is a case of complete deafness and dumbness cured by mesmerism, as presented by Dr. John Elliotson.

On the 25th of April, 1840, a very poor boy, fifteen years of age, tall and strong, named Thomas Russen, completely deaf and dumb, was brought to me by his father, with a note from a lady at Twickenham, a stranger to me, requesting I would take pity upon him and endeavor to cure him. She had herself, she said, been a witness to the wonderful cure of Master Linell.

According to the boy's father, the youngster lived with him at Twickenham and supported himself by fetching small periodicals twice a week from London, distributing them in the neighborhood. On the first of April he had gone as usual to Number 4 Bridgers Street, Covent Gardens, for books and newspapers, and had to procure four dozen Loyds Weekly London Newspaper. Accidentally, the boy forgot two dozen of the newspapers, discovering the loss when he arrived home. When his father returned home he scolded the lad, accusing him of spending the money on liquor.

Father and son walked to Richmond and the boy got an omnibus to London, hoping to find the lost newspapers where he had left them. He remembers nothing more after this than that he one day "awoke as from a deep sleep in a strange place, began looking around him, tried in vain to speak, and could not hear any noise at all. Seeing a board over the fireplace with the words 'King's College Hospital' upon it, he learnt where he was."

The father ascertained that when his son returned to the newspaper office he found that his papers had been carried off by someone, and no more were to be had til the next day. Then the boy had gone to a neighboring coffee house and had been seized by a most violent epileptic fit, and was carried by the police to the King's College Hospital, where he lay perfectly insensible for four days and five nights.

The following is extracted from an account which the boy wrote out for me after his recovery:

Then I knew where I was and found that all was very quiet and I tried to speak and could not. And when the doctors came they asked me a great many questions (written out), and Dr. Guy asked me if I ever had the hands passed before my eyes, and I told him no. And when the students came they began asking me such foolish questions. One was, Does your mother know you're out? And this is my answer—That is joking, but still she knows that I am not at home now. Another question: Have you ever been in the same way before? And I answered, I have had fits but not been so bad before. . . . And then Dr. Todd hallowed in my ear, and asked me if I had felt it, and I told him that I heard a noise, like a pot boiling. And a great many other foolish questions they asked me. And a young man in the hospital told me that Dr. Todd said "cuckoo" in my ear, and then they wrote down that I should not have any food til I spoke and asked them for some; but they gave me some when I told them I could not ask for any. One day Dr. Budd saw me and said, Oh, the damn young scoundrel, he is only shamming. If I were Dr. Todd I would whip him until he did speak! That's what the Sister told me. She wrote it down. And when Dr. Todd came I told him, and he told me to take off my jacket and shirt, and he would give me the whip. And I did take them off, but he did not whip me. And then he ordered me a cold shower bath every morning, and I had it five times. And one day, when father came to see me, Dr. Russel, the house surgeon, told him that it was of no use keeping me there any longer. So father brought me out with him, after I had been in 21 days. I do not know what they did to me when there, during the time I was insensible, which was four days and five nights; only, a young man, a patient in the hospital, told me that they thrust pins in me and burnt me with hot spoons and did several other things to me as well, to make me speak.

It required very little sagacity to know in five minutes that the boy was completely deaf and dumb. He could not hear the loudest or shrillest sound, or make any noise above the faintest puff, or mere breath sound, however forcibly he expired. I subsequently learned that he had been seized several times over the past four years with violent epileptic fits.

I determined on doing what I could for him with mesmerism. Standing before him I made slow passes downwards before his face and, after a time, merely pointed the fingers of one hand to his eyes. The former had no sensible effect, but when I merely pointed, his eyelids began to wink and continued winking more and more strongly to the end of the half hour, which I resolved to devote to him.

The next day and ever afterwards the eyes began winking as soon as I pointed to them. The winking became stronger, and the itching and smarting of the eyes obliged him to rub them. The eyes began closing, and after a few days the eyes continued closed for some moments—there being evidently snatches of sleep.

The effect was invariably less the instant I changed the pointing to passes, and soon ceased altogether. The periods of sleep lasted longer and longer. In a fortnight I had only to point to his eyes, two or three seconds, and he always dropped into the profoundest sleep.

I was too busy for two or three days to do more than send him to sleep and trust to the general influence of mesmerism for the local benefit. On the third day I pointed my fingers into both his ears for some time during his sleep, and he then began to express pain in and around them as he slept. In two days more the pain was felt at various hours when he was awake and rapidly increased, til at the beginning of the next week it was dreadful. And when I had put him to sleep he not only put his hands to his ears, but struck them violently, drew up his legs and kicked, struck his head against the wall. The tears rolled copiously down his cheeks, his face was flushed, and he sometimes was almost frantic, but made not the faintest noise all this time, nor did he awake.

I was obliged at last to lay him on the floor in his sleep. The pains agonized him in the waking state, and it was distressing to see him come to me every morning with his cheeks flushed, his eyes red with crying, his cheeks wet with tears, his handkerchief in his hand, and his countenance expressive of the most intense suffering. He walked from beyond Twickenham and back every day—a distance altogether of twenty-two miles. He had become so susceptible that pointing at him, even with anything, or staring at him, immediately made his eyelids quiver and in two moments always sent him into his deep sleep, which however did not last above a quarter of an hour or twenty minutes.

On May 17th, a day or two before the pains were evident, and three days before I put my fingers into his ears, while asleep he appeared to dream, held up one finger and inclined his head forward and a little sideways, in the most natural and therefore beautiful attitude of that of listening for a short time. On the third day of the week in which his pain had become so severe, I resolved to bestow more time on him. As he lay on the floor, several gentlemen being in the room, I sat behind his head, held it raised as well as I could, and inserted the extremities of my forefingers into his ears. This was rather troublesome to continue, as he tossed his head in all directions, and struck his arms and legs about from time to time in agony. At last he awoke, and on my making some observations he smiled—*he had recovered his hearing.* But he could not utter a sound.

I sent him to sleep again and kept the points of all my fingers under the front of his lower jaw, against the root of his tongue and his larynx, at the top of the windpipe. After a time he began to make efforts to speak. The root of the tongue and the larynx began moving, and the former swelling. At length an expiratory sound was audible—louder than the faint breathing sound hitherto heard when he strained to make a noise. I persevered with my fingers and his efforts increased. The sound augmented, actually becoming strong, and then he half articulated, and at last spoke perfectly well, waking in the midst of his efforts.

The joy of all present can be imagined. Mr. Thomas walked across the room, shook my hand in the warmth of his heart, and the next day provided for the boy by taking him into his establishment in Yorkshire.

Case 8: Hysterical Epilepsy

This is a case of hysterical epilepsy presented by Dr. John Elliotson.

In December 1839, I was requested by Mr. Hallion of Warren Street to see a young lady named Spong, residing at 31 High Street, Camdentown. She was sixteen years old and lying on her back upon a machine, on account of a curvature of her spine, and had severe epileptic fits with some symptoms of hysteria.

She had enjoyed good health until her thirteenth year, when, in the spring of 1836, she frequently fainted and had a pain in her left side and her spine became curved. In November of the same year the faintings changed to epileptic fits. She was placed upon her back on an apparatus, under the care of Mr. Thornber, but the epileptic fits were so violent that the cure was prevented, and Mr. Thornber wished to give up the case.

She required five people to hold her, and in spite of them all would turn round on her face. Mr. Carter, now of Redding and then Mr. Hallion mesmerised her twice a week for six months. Her fits continued as frequent as before, but were less violent so that she did not require holding and was not exhausted as previously on coming out of them. She fell asleep when mesmerised for a quarter of an hour.

I mesmerised her in December 1839, and she went to sleep the first time. I spoke to her and she answered me and proved to be in the deeper sleep-waking, and knew me and knew she was asleep. I asked whether I should be able to cure her. "Yes." I inquired when: "In four months."*

Her attacks were numerous and in rapid succession when they came upon her. Originally they came every other day for six months, then once a week, and for six months on a Tuesday at the same hour, then once a fortnight for the last two years. She had taken medicine all along, but in vain. Her face was always so swollen and red the next day that she could not be seen.

She predicted to me not only the period of their cessation, *but the day and hour of each attack*. She said the next would be on Thursday, and her mother could scarcely believe her senses when she saw them come on that day. They returned about once a fortnight, on no regular day or hour, but always as she foretold to me in the mesmeric sleep-waking.

She opened her eyes at my bidding, but no attempt at tractive or other experiments succeeded and no other powers were developed. I mesmerised her twice a week for a month, and then only once a fortnight when the attack was expected, during the attack, and after it was over. Mr. Hallion also, however, mesmerised her twice a week. She had nine fits every attack, except the last, and then she had only one—exactly as predicted.

Trusting to her prediction, I discontinued the mesmerism when the four months were expired, *and the disease has never returned*.

Case 9: Intense Hiccough

On the evening of Friday, January 4, 1839, a fortnight after I had resigned my office of Professor in University College, London, because the Council, at the instigation of the

---

*This is another instance of prognostication which proved true.

medical professors, in cooperation with Mr. Wakley (editor of the *Lancet*) forbade that any cures should be effected with mesmerism in the hospital, I was called upon by Mr. Johnstone of 22 Saville Row to a young lady rather about twenty years of age, who had been seized that very evening with the severest hiccough I ever witnessed.

On the 22nd of December some friends fired off a pistol for "fun" in the room where she was. A young man, having a short time previously said that he would shoot her through the window, she at the moment supposed she was shot. Immediately she was seized with a violent, hard, dry, barking, ringing cough. It grew worse and worse, and on the 25th Mr. Johnstone was called in. He bled her twice in the arm, blistered her chest, and gave her various medicines. But the cough continued to grow worse and worse. On January 4th, after she had complained of sickness all day, it suddenly changed in the evening to an equally severe hiccough.

I shall be pardoned for making two remarks here: the first that of all cruel absurdities, to frighten others unnecessarily is the worst. I have attended so many cases of St. Vitus' dance, epilepsy, insanity, fatuity, palsy, et cetera, from terror in sport, that the danger of terror cannot be too generally known, nor the duty too strongly inculcated of abstaining from tricks intended to produce it, and from supplying children with the superstitious, and therefore detestable, ideas of the existence of goblins, evil spirits, and the reality of the mythos of the devil. The second remark is that the spasmodic, nervous cough, which preceded the hiccough in this case, and is so rebellious to all the established modes of treatment, usually yields to mesmerism as its proper remedy.

Not knowing at that time the superiority of Mr. Johnstone's character, but knowing the complete ignorance and the irrational and coarse feeling of the medical profession at large in reference to mesmerism, and well aware of the equally gross ignorance and prejudice of the public—fostered so assiduously by medical men—I did not mention mesmerism, presuming it would be rejected. However, without any remark I proceeded as if to press the pit of the stomach in the ordinary way under the bedclothes with one hand. But I took the opportunity of *pointing my fingers upon it* and keeping them there for some minutes. The effect of this little mesmeric proceeding was that the hiccough ceased for an hour. This I learnt at my visit the next morning when, however, she was as bad as ever.

I could not refrain now from telling Mr. Johnstone what I had done. But it appears that I mentioned merely having placed my hand upon the pit of the stomach, for Mr. Johnstone did not understand me to have done more. He very liberally tried the plan, but with no advantage. The patient long afterwards told us that I *pointed my fingers,* and she felt great relief, but that Mr. Johnstone *applied his hand,* and she felt no relief. This little incident is well worth attention.

In February, six weeks after I had seen her, Dr. Chowne of Charing Cross Hospital was called in. He prescribed a compound-iron mixture, ammonia, camphor, and a tincture. The disease went on, increasing all this time, reducing her strength more and more. Those who have experienced a very strong hiccough, an hour or two after dinner, know how distressing and painful it is, but still can form no idea of the violence and agony of this case. The straining was as if she were being torn asunder, and always ending in vomiting, which would bring up things taken twelve hours before. It rolled her in her bed and raised her so that, but for her attendants, she would have been thrown off, and she entreated them to hold her down.

The gulping noise of the spasms, when the streets were quiet, was heard even in Regeant Street. Her only respite was obtained by lying perfectly flat and perfectly still—all noise in the room being at the same time avoided.

However motionless she remained, a knock at the door, the least noise in the room, nay, the presence of more than two persons in the room brought on the attack. And during the hiccough—however many hours it lasted—to take food was impossible. After a severe attack she would be unable to speak for hours, or even to swallow, and could not bear the weight of the bedclothes. She was always cold, whatever number of blankets were heaped upon her. No action of the bowels occurred without aperients. It was feared that nature could not hold out much longer, when mesmerism was suggested.

The patient and her family did not know exactly what was meant by mesmerism, and Mr. Johnstone was asked his opinion of it. Very greatly to his credit, Mr. Johnstone, while he confessed that he knew almost nothing of mesmerism, though he had seen singular effects apparently produced by it, and had laughed at it like others, said that, everything else having failed, he saw no objection to a trial of it, and offered to consult me upon the point.

How different was this conduct from that of many who fancied themselves great doctors and surgeons, and liberal intellectuals and philosophical, "enlightened members of an honorable profession" with "a high moral feeling."

Accordingly, on the morning of February 27, 1839, I seated myself by the side of her couch and began to make slow passes down before her face. She had no idea of what I was doing, or what effect could possibly be expected. After twenty minutes her eyes closed and could not be opened, til at the end of the sitting I rubbed my thumbs outwards upon the eyebrows. Her mouth nearly closed and her speech became indistinct. The hiccough—which the idea of being mesmerised in the presence of four or five persons had excited—gradually subsided as I went on.

At the end of half an hour the doorbell suddenly rang, but produced no hiccough, as it invariably had up to that time. I now tried the effect of raising her by winding up that movable part of the couch, and thus brought on the hiccough, which, however, ceased as soon as she was lowered again and mesmerised afresh. This second mesmerisation produced the same effects as the first. I rubbed her eyebrows as before. Her eyes opened, and I left her. She had no other attack the rest of the day and was quite cheerful.

February 28: Her eyes closed in a few minutes and could not be opened by any other person than myself, rubbing the eyebrows outwards. At the end of half an hour, besides the rigid closure of the eyes and stiffness of the jaw, there was a certain stiffness of the whole body, with a feeling of stupidity* and of constriction of the chest. The hiccough—which, as on the day before, had begun from the idea of being mesmerised—soon subsided. And I actually raised her, and I moved her up and down several times without producing the hiccough. She now felt warm and comfortable, which she never had before.

March 1: Her eyes and mouth closed and her whole body stiffened; her arms became rather stiff; she felt stupid, but did not lose herself. I raised her again and again without producing hiccough, and she had suffered no hiccough all day. After I was gone she kept raised for twenty minutes, and only a slight hiccough was occasioned, which however ceased as soon as she was laid down. She was better all the evening.

I continued to mesmerise this patient every day. The

---

*The word "stupidity" is used in the sense of "dullness."

eyes always closed firmly, then at length the jaw. The body became more and more rigid and the arms and legs became rigid likewise, but the legs grew rigid the last. Just as at each mesmerisation *the effects began in the eyes and gradually descended,* so the degree of the effects increased in the course of the mesmeric treatment. . . . at the end of ten days she walked six steps with the effect of only a very slight hiccough.

At length the rigidity extended to her legs and, though on the 30th of March they were strong enough to support her in the sleep-waking state without assistance, they were incapable of walking or advancing a hair's breadth.

The stupidity went on to perfect sleep, and the disease presently ceased. In a fortnight from the commencement of the mesmerism she could bear to be dressed. She slept well without narcotics, which previously had been required every night. She was warm, whereas before during the whole of her illness she had been distressingly cold. She could eat, and did eat well, and recovered her strength and plumpness, and astonished all her friends—and this without a particle of medicine.

Case 10: Treatment of Injured Horses

The charge was often leveled at those who practiced Animal Magnetism that the patients were "shamming" or "faking" their diseases. Dr. Elliotson and his colleagues suffered constantly from malicious gossip and slander which sought to destroy their research and their efforts. It is always easier to cry "fake!" than it is to investigate work in basically new fields of discovery.

Following are two short cases of the use of Animal Magnetism on two horses in Dr. Elliotson's stables. Certainly, the ability of a horse "to cure himself" or indulge in "fakery" would seem even more incredible than the results gained through the use of Animal Magnetism.

Last winter (1844) I tried the power of mesmerism in inflammation on two horses. The first had fallen in the stall and had severely injured his eye. There was great inflammation. The eyelids were closed and very much swollen, and the eye seemed seriously injured. The cornea was quite opaque.

I mesmerised the eye by passes over it for half an hour, when the animal opened the eye and the inflammation was considerably abated. The first ten minutes the horse did not seem to experience any sensation. Afterwards, however, it was evident that it did so, as it slightly twitched its head away every time I passed my hand over the eye—although I did not touch it but made the passes at a few inches distance.

The operation was repeated by my groom that day, and twice the following day, when all swelling had subsided and there was no sign of inflammation, merely a white streak across the cornea, evidently from the severity of the blow. It was some months before this streak was quite obliterated. No other means were used at all for the animal's recovery.

The second case was that of a horse who had a severe cut on the back sinew of the foreleg. There was a great inflammation in the leg, and the horse, from pain, had not placed its foot firmly on the ground from a few hours after the accident. On the third day I made passes down the leg at the distance of about one inch from the leg. I continued the process for little more than half an hour, when the leg was considerably cooler, and the horse placed the foot flat and firmly on the ground. I have tried no other experiments of this kind on brutes.

Case 11: Enlarged Glands

NOTE: *This case, as well as the succeeding seven cases, was reported to Dr. Elliotson by Dr. James Esdaile, a brilliant physician and surgeon, who directed the Mesmeric Hospital of Calcutta, India. Dr. Esdaile is best known for his superb success using Animal Magnetism as the only anesthetic in hundreds of major surgical operations. Less well known are the nonsurgical cases, some of which are presented here.*

Miss Gordon, an East Indian by birth, age 18, of lymphatic temperament, has been suffering for two years from enlargement of the glands of the throat and neck, extending from the ear to the shoulder. The disfigurement is very great. Her gland at the angle of the jaw is as big as an egg, and the chain from the ear to the shoulder is raised to the thickness of three fingers, impeding all motion on that side. There are also single enlarged glands in the upper triangle of the neck, and one in the lower as big as a large marble. Tenderness on pressure is very considerable in most of the glands and they are all extremely hard. She has derived no benefit from medical treatment under different doctors.

January 18, 1846: She has been mesmerized (for approximately three weeks now) daily, both locally and generally. The swellings are sensibly softer and somewhat reduced in size.

January 29: She has occasionally gone to sleep and generally feels drowsy under the process. The swellings are reduced to a remarkable degree, and a third part only remains near the angle of the jaw. The lower portion that prevented nearly all motion, has disappeared, and she moves her head with a little impediment to that side. The single glands in the triangle of the neck have nearly disappeared and there is every prospect of the whole being speedily absorbed.

Case 12: Rheumatic Lameness

Mouli Mahmud, a boatman age 30, a native of Chitigang, admitted to the hospital January 14, 1847, has been troubled with rheumatism for five years. It was attended with fever every evening for the first three or four months.

All the articulations of the joints are more or less painful, but especially those of the ankles, knees, wrists, and fingers. The ankles are considerably swollen and exceedingly tender to the touch, and there is much pain in one heel. For a month past he cannot walk without the support of a staff. He is to be mesmerized locally and generally for an hour daily.

No remarkable change was perceived during the first four days of mesmerizing, except that the pains became more general and the joints easier.

January 20: He sleeps at the time of mesmerizing, and now and then is put to sleep by the local process alone. The swelling and pain of the joints are much diminished. He allows them to be handled freely, excepting the ankles, which are still slightly swollen and painful. He can walk out of the room without his stick.

January 23: He has no pain in the joints. He can move them without pain. He walks about without his stick but limps a little.

January 25: He feels quite well and has no pain in the ankles. He walks, runs, and leaps without the least pain, and was discharged today at his own request, quite well.

Case 13: Chronic Rheumatism and Stiff Elbow Joints

Mr. de Broulet, a Frenchman, merchant in Calcutta, age 32, has been suffering from rheumatism for the last six months. His left elbow is much enlarged, very tender and stiff—it is half bent and can neither be bent nor extended. Numerous enlarged glands surround the joint and the least

Numerous enlarged glands surround the joint and the least pressure is exquisitely painful. The wrist is also quite stiff. The other elbow is a little contracted and painful, but not enlarged, and there are two unhealthy abscesses at the top of the breast bone where the surrounding parts are swollen and very tender.

The left elbow is scarred all over by blisters and cauteries, from which he derived no benefit, and he has abandoned all medical treatment. His nights are very restless, and he can with great difficulty turn himself in bed. He cannot without help take off or put on his coat. His spirits and appetite are bad, and his nervous system is much broken. He is to come to the hospital daily for an hour, to be mesmerized locally and generally.

January 16: The abscesses were opened today and a quantity of unhealthy matter let out.

January 18: He slept during the mesmerizing yesterday and had a good night afterwards. Today the pains are much less.

January 20: He can move the left wrist freely. The pain in the elbow joint is much less, and he can dress himself without help.

January 25: Nearly all pain has disappeared from the left elbow, and he can bear it to be freely pressed and even struck with little pain, and can bend it nearly to the natural degree, and the wrist is quite free. He sleeps well. His spirits and appetite are much improved. He has slept daily during the last week of the mesmerizing and bears considerable extension of the arm without waking. On several occasions he has tried to keep awake to witness certain experiments that were going on in the room, but found it to be impossible. The pain and enlargement around the sores on his breast are nearly gone.

January 27: I worked his elbow with considerable force

today when he was asleep. There is enlargement of the ends of the bone and grating about the joints, and the head of the radius is impacted by morbid adhesions. He was not aware of this rough treatment on waking. It is clear the impediment to motion now is purely mechanical and will probably be overcome to a great degree by time and exercise. The original inflammation is extinguished.

Case 14: Paralysis

A peddler, residing in Calcutta, has been suffering for about sixteen days with hemiplegia.* The illness came on in the course of a single night. He went to bed in perfect good health and found the whole of the left side of his body totally paralyzed next morning. There is a complete palsy of all the left side. The left fist is firmly clenched and cannot be opened without much difficulty. The left side of his face is permanently distorted and drawn upwards. The left foot and leg are rigidly extended. The left side of the tongue is also paralyzed, and he can utter only indistinct sounds, which he does with great exertion. He falls to the ground like a wet rag when not supported, and when made to sit up he falls over to the left side like a dead body when support is removed. He is to be mesmerized for an hour daily.

April 8 (1847): He did not sleep at the time of being mesmerized.

April 11: He can raise the forearm and the leg considerably from the bed and slightly open his hand. The spasm of the face is much abated and the distortion can hardly be recognized.

April 13: He can sit up and speak pretty distinctly. He has so far regained the use of the affected limb that he can make it partially bear the weight of his body in the act of walking with a slight support.

---

*Paralysis of only one-half of the body.

April 18: He got up from bed and walked in the room with a staff today. He could stand even without it. He complained of spasm and pain in the affected side.

April 24: He is getting stronger daily in the affected limbs. The spasm of the parts is nearly gone. He now walks without a staff and can raise the paralyzed arm considerably but cannot open or close the fist.

April 27: He slept in the open veranda and exposed himself to the cold air and became worse. His voice became hoarse, and the affected side was felt heavier and lost in some measure the vitality which had been restored. He coughs and cannot expectorate. To have one-half ounce of cough mixture thrice a day. He is not able to arise from his bed, and in attempting to do so tumbled down.

May 1: He appears a little better, regaining strength in the leg, but the arm cannot be moved, raised or bent. The fist remains closed, but can be easily extended.

May 7: He walks without a staff, and the limb affords considerable resistance at the time. He can bend, extend, and raise the forearm. He feels much aching in the affected side and breathes much freer. His voice is improved.

May 21: He can bend and extend the leg pretty freely. It bears the weight of his body with great firmness. He can raise and bend the arm much better. He is getting strength daily in the affected side and walks safely about the compound. He begged leave to go and see his family for a day but promised to return. If he does his case will be continued.

Case 15: Ulcers of the Head

Following is a statement written by Mary Ford (Mrs. G. Ford) to the physician, following her treatment with mesmerism:

My health declined more than ten years ago. I have been

afflicted with violent pains in the head, with burning feet, pains in my temples and way over my eyes—worse always at night. It [the pain] will be a month or six weeks gathering, being very sore and bad to bear, then the places will break and discharge, more like hot water when it first breaks than when it has kept running for a long time. It has run more than two years at once. Since then I have had three broken places in my head and two in my forehead. I have been under several doctors at the hospital and several out. They have said it was not 'the evil,' but have never said what it was.

"I have been very poorly in my health, scarcely able to do for myself and for my family. I have been ordered to use bread poultices, linseed poultices, ointments and lotions at different times. I have been to the Dispensary to the Canterbury Hospital.

"I think it was in February you, sir, took me in hand. And I can say for a truth you have done me more good than all the doctors I have been under, for which I feel thankful to God for that He put it into your heart to do me so much good. And I can say from my very heart, I have great cause to be thankful.

(signed) Mary Ford

Following are the notes of the operator in this case:

February 29, 1848: Commenced to mesmerize Mrs. G. Ford, who for ten years has had ulcers on her head. One of them has penetrated almost through the skull. She is pale, weak, and seemingly sinking. She went into sleep-waking in a few seconds.

March 1: Mrs. Ford informed me that she had passed a good night, free from pain, and that the pain in her head, which was relieved yesterday, has not returned. She said that she had not been able for a long time to sleep on the left side of her head where there is a bad ulcer, but that last night she did so with comfort.

March 2: Mrs. Ford had pain in her head when she came this morning, which was soon relieved. She told me that she has long been accustomed to moan in the night from the pain and the dizziness in her head, but that this morning her husband said to her, "Why, you did not grunt in the night."

"No," she replied, "I had no need to grunt." She passed an easy night.

March 3: Mrs. Ford has had another good night and says she feels better. The ulcers are beginning to get drier. I examined them this morning. The large ulcer appears to penetrate nearly to the brain, for there is a hole almost through the skull.

March 4: During sleep-waking this morning, Mrs. Ford had, what she has been long accustomed to, a painful spasm in her throat. Not being able to describe her sensations, she became alarmed and nervous, and after she awoke was a little hysterical. It soon, however, passed off.

March 6: In order to avoid a recurrence of this spasm in the throat, I kept Mrs. Ford a shorter time in sleep-waking, which was very quiet and refreshing to her.

March 7: Very quiet today and no return of unpleasant symptoms. She slept well, has quite lost the pain in her head, and can sleep equally well on either side of it. She considers herself very much better.

March 17: With one or two exceptions, I have mesmerized Mrs. G. Ford every day and she has uniformly slept well. She gains strength, sleeps quietly, is quite free from pain, *and all the wounds in her head have dried up.*

March 18: Mrs. Ford had the last sitting this morning. She says she feels quite well. She has not been so well for years and does not wish to feel better. She has a healthy color. When dismissed from the hospital she has always been dismissed as "relieved," never as cured. Now at present she announces herself to be "quite well."

Case 16: Lumbar Abscess and Disease of the Spine

Dr. John Elliotson presents the following case, remarking: "Here is another cure of a disease, not at all of the nervous system, and without the possibility of ascription to imagination."

I was consulted respecting a little boy deformed in his back, bent forward with his hands on his knees and an evident large collection of matter in his loins, pale with a hectic flush, emaciated and feeble. I gave no hope, for I had never seen a recovery from such a state of things.

When afterwards I was questioned respecting the utility of mesmerism in this case, I replied that I certainly would recommend a good persevering trial of it, because I was continually seeing it affect cures which absolutely astonished me and which nothing else could; and because I felt certain that no medicine, nothing in the routines of physics or surgery could save his life. Mesmerism I knew would support his strength and might enable Nature to get the better of the disease. I subjoin the father's simple story of the cure.

(The following history was written by James Davis Horn of Coursham.)

In the summer of 1845, my son, Michael Ford Horn, nine years of age, had a fall and soon after complained of a pain in his back. In the month of December a bone appeared to be growing out, and we observed a swelling in his back. And in the beginning of January 1846 I took him to Mr. Norman of Bath, who pronounced the disease to be a lumbar abscess and said he scarcely ever knew a person to recover from one. Mr. Norman told me it would continue to increase in size until it broke, and then it would "run him out"—that he might, however, live for two years, but that it would ultimately cause his death. Mr. Norman saw him after this, three or four times, and still expressed the same opinion.

I was ordered by Mr. Norman to let him lie in bed, and Mr. Norman prescribed some strengthening powders and a box of ointment.

My son remained till the month of May still getting

worse. At this time he could not walk more than twenty yards at a time, and then only by placing his hands upon his knees. I soon after heard from Mr. Valance of Bristol that Dr. Harrup at Brighton was very skillful, had affected many cures of spinal diseases and, amongst others, in one of his own family.

I took my child to Brighton and showed him to Dr. Harrup, who said it was a blood tumor and he would not survive long. I then with a heavy heart returned to London on my way home. But my brother who resides there wished me to have further advice. So we took him to Dr. Elliotson, who likewise told me it was a hopeless case of diseased spine and lumbar abscess.* I must not forget to speak of the kindness of both the last-mentioned gentlemen, who refused to accept of any fee.

The next day I returned home with my child, without the smallest hope of recovery. I received a letter from my brother stating that a friend of his had advised mesmerism be tried. I knew nothing about mesmerism, but anxious to avail myself of anything that promised relief to my dear child, I again returned to London. This friend called immediately at my brother's and made passes for about a half an hour daily without producing sleep. He was anxious that sleep should be produced before I left London, that I might have confidence to proceed myself on my return to the country, and with this view recommended me to Mr. Decimus Hands of Thayer Street, Manchester Square, who mesmerized him daily for some weeks. But after a week or two no attempt was made to produce sleep—*the passes being made over the abscess.*

While under Mr. Hands' care, the abscess broke and dis-

---

*A most interesting aspect of this case is that Dr. Elliotson himself thought the case so hopeless that he did not even attempt to employ Animal Magnetism on the child.

charged upwards of a quart of matter. The mesmerism was still continued and the child remained about the same in regard to his health. During his stay in London, he was seen several times by Earl Doucey, who took a kind interest in him, Mr. Highet, MP, Captain James and Major Buckley. Dr. Elliotson advised me to persevere with mesmerism, because, though he feared it would fail, still there was no other remedy.

Some time after this, Mr. Hands' health compelled him to go into the country, and I therefore took the child home and continued the passes myself. The third day of my attempt, the mesmeric sleep was produced, and I continued to produce the sleep daily until the following spring. It appeared that when in London it was prevented by his fear lest if he went to sleep an operation would be performed upon him.

Some time after he returned home another abscess formed in the back, broke, and discharged a great quantity of matter, and the child was very much reduced, not being able to move. He was in such a dreadful state that I began to despair of saving him, but I was induced to persevere with the mesmerism, and truly thankful I am that I did so.

The second abscess broke in November 1846, and in February 1847 a decided improvement was perceived. From that time the child continued to mend rapidly. By still continuing my exertions, he gained strength and has continued to do so to the present time. The abscesses are, I may say, healed, for there is scarcely a stain upon his linen—and the child is running about from morning till night in perfect health and quite straight.

He has not taken any medicine whatever during all this time. I attribute his cure entirely under the blessing of God to mesmerism.

(signed) James Davis Horn
Coursham, Wilts.

In the light of this extraordinary case, and in view of the fact that traditional medicine held no hope out for this child, the following opinions by orthodox science appear as spiteful as they are malicious:

> Do not quacks hunt out the vices or infirmities of mankind to turn them to profit, some selecting one and some another for their purpose. Among quacks, the impostors called 'mesmerists' are in my opinion the especial favorites of those, both male and female, in whom the sexual passions burn strongly, either in secret or notoriously. Decency forbids me to be more explicit. . . . (From an oration delivered by Dr. F. Hawkins before the London College of Physicians, June 24, 1848)

The viciousness of the above quotation is equalled, if not exceeded, by another mortal enemy of mesmerism:

> With every respect for the vast extent of human credulity, we do think that the brood of mesmerism are its own natural and most powerful enemies, and that they must in time utterly destroy their loathsome dam. (Mr. Wakley, editor of *The Lancet,* July 8, 1848)

Case 17: Insanity

In writing up this case, Dr. John Elliotson hits back at his detractors, who, like secret moles, were forever undermining his reputation and his work. The case follows:

In November 1842, Mr. Morgan, surgeon of Bedford Row, called on me to request if I would see a poor child whom he had been treating for four months without the least benefit, and in whose case no measures of the ordinary routine of medicine now suggested themselves to him as calculated to be of any use.

The child's mother had heard of the mesmeric treatment and asked him to go to me to try to cure the child with mesmerism.

Mr. Morgan did not sail in a passion at the woman for her "ignorance and impudence." He neither swore nor bounced; neither did he laugh at her as a fool! He did not tell her that "mesmerism was a complete humbug and wonder how she could believe in such nonsense! He did not tell her that I "was a quack—a very clever man *once*, but now a lost man!" He did not say that I was mad, that "nobody now cared what I said," that "Mr. Wakley had exposed all mesmerists and mesmeric patients and destroyed mesmerism years ago forever!"

He did not tell this mother that I "had been turned out of University College and its hospital on account of prescribing mesmerism," and that "Dr. Forbes had killed mesmerism after Mr. Wakley had killed it, and both would kill it several times yet!" He did not add that my prospects were ruined, that I "was ruined and going to leave England forever!" He did not tell her that "mesmerism was a most dangerous thing, and persons could not sometimes be awakened again, and that it might cause apoplexy and perhaps insanity for life!"

He did not threaten that if the child was mesmerized— though he confessed he could do nothing for it and was no longer attempting to do anything for it—he would "never attend it again!" And, "should the mother have any more family, that he would not attend her in her confinement if mesmerism were allowed to enter the house!" All which deliberate falsehoods and threats have come to my knowledge as uttered by modern practitioners of what is absurdly called "high-standing and middle-standing Royal Practitioners," "titled Practitioners," "graduates of English Universities, Fellows of Colleges, Hospital Physicians and Surgeons, and Professors and Teachers"!

Mr. Morgan did not say to this mother, as the most fashionable physician of the hour did to a Baronet—a patient of mine who consulted him in my absence—"Oh, that gentleman who has always got some crotchet or other and has now got hold of mesmerism." And on being asked if he had ever witnessed a mesmeric case replied: "No, and nothing shall ever induce me!"

No—Mr. Morgan immediately called upon me and made the request, honestly saying (and I use the words of a letter subsequently written to me by him): "Certain it is that neither myself nor others have produced the least benefit upon a set of symptoms as strange as I ever witnessed and as difficult to me at least to understand or describe."

Mr. Morgan's letter continues: "In the summer of 1842 I first saw her laboring under the following symptoms: constant pain in her head; she was with difficulty roused to the slightest exertion; bowels obstinately caustic; lying for weeks in a semi-comatose state, sometimes crying, again laughing, painfully susceptible to the least noise. At one time refusing food, at another ravenous. . . . I was at a loss what to do and sent for you."

On the fourth of November, 1842, at four o'clock in the afternoon, I accordingly went to see the child. Her name was Sarah Wiltshire, and her age, eleven years. The account given by the mother was the following: She (the mother) herself had been attacked in the mews by a drunken man who abused her in the grossest manner. The child (who apparently witnessed the event) was terrified, seized with a violent tremor, screamed excessively and continued to do so. At length her hands became clenched, her jaws locked, and she fell into insensibility, which lasted three days, her head working about all the time, and not a particle of food or drink being swallowed. Her sensibility then returned and she ate voraciously, lying constantly on her back, moaning, rolling her head and working her hands. A fit of screaming and rage took place every hour or two in which she attempted to bite everybody.

The bowels were never relieved without medicine, and she had also a violent cough, like the barking of a dog. In this state I now beheld the child. She could not speak and had not spoken from the first, and the bowels had not acted for nine days, nor had she slept an hour at a time. She was pale and looked thin, sickly, and fatuitous, and would not sit up in bed.

Thus, there was extreme general debility and the greater part of the nervous system was in disorder. She was fatuitous and maniacal. Finding that aperients—like all other medical means—had failed, and what was worse, had always aggravated the symptoms, I entreated that no aperients, nor indeed any other drugs should be given, whatever length of time the bowels might remain torpid.

I have repeatedly seen the cure of St. Vitus' dance thrown back by the use of active purgatives or by diarrhea excited by eating improper things while the disease was yielding to iron, with which I have never failed to cure the disease when I superintended its use myself. Feeble, nervous, and dyspeptic persons suffer exceedingly similar injudicious treatment as well as by the prevalent use of mercury. Many such patients are the better for habitual action (of the bowels) but once every second or third day.

I made slow and long passes at a very short distance from her, from opposite the forehead to opposite the stomach as she lay. At first she continued moving her head about and away from me, moaning and very cross, and she never fixed her eyes upon me or anything. But in twenty minutes she was fast asleep. Her head ceased to roll and the moaning was no longer heard. On my speaking to her she was roused up, but a repetition of the passes for five minutes sent her back into sleep as sound as ever. And I left her asleep, silent and motionless. It was now twenty minutes to five, and I desired that she might be undisturbed and allowed to awake spontaneously. She slept from that time till two o'clock in the morning—*about nine hours*—she who had not slept one hour together for the previous ten weeks!

Was all this "fear-induced imposture?" Was her disease "imposture"? Was the deep trance, the stillness of head and hands, the silence of more than nine hours the "result of imagination" in this poor, violent and fatuitous object? Was it [as detractors claimed] "Manchester fatigue" of her eyes? Mr. Wood visited the patient daily and continued what I had begun.

November 5: Sent again to sleep and left sleepy. She had not screamed from the time she was mesmerized yesterday, and though she was left sleepy only, she slept well all night and is altogether better.

November 6: The head was rolling about as usual but became quiet as soon as mesmerization was begun, and she was soon asleep.

November 7: Slept from the time she was mesmerized yesterday at 6 P.M., until 4 A.M.—ten hours, when she woke for a few minutes and slept again til 6 A.M., making it twelve hours. She also slept on her side for the first time since the seizure four months before. The cough, which had been very troublesome, was also greatly reduced. She had recovered her speech, but it was only to use bad and violent language to all about her in the fits of frenzy which often seized her. She was mesmerized in the afternoon and left asleep.

November 8: She slept from the afternoon of yesterday til 8 A.M. today. During the mesmerization today the cough ceased. She turned on her left side and went to sleep and was left sleeping. Her bowels acted today spontaneously.

November 9: She slept from 6 P.M. last evening til 7 this morning—thirteen hours. She had no cough today, is stronger and decidedly better.

November 16: [The patient was given purgatives, despite

Dr. Elliotson's warnings that she should be given none.]
Symptoms are much aggravated and she is much weaker. I
have often observed that the effects of causes injurious to
health are felt, as in this instance, more afterwards than immediately.

November 17: She slept for a short time only, was left
asleep, and she seems to be nearly as bad as before she was
mesmerized. Mesmerism has thus had far less power over her
now she was reduced [by the purgatives]. I have often been
unable to produce any appreciable effect upon extremely
weak persons, even when their complaints were seated in
the nervous system and they were exceedingly nervous. . . .
weakness does not favor mesmeric susceptibility.*

November 18: She slept longer and is much stronger.

November 19 to December 3: Sleeps well at night; still
improving.

December 10: Much better, but still rolls her head.

December 16: Stronger. Spasmodic cough gone.

January 20: No symptoms, but a degree of debility. Will
be mesmerised but twice a week.

February 1: Perfectly well and walks about as usual. To
be mesmerized but once a week. Her bowels always act
regularly.

Mesmerism was discontinued on February 20th. In the
autumn, seven months after her cure, she was terrified by the
same man and suffered a relapse, which, however, was soon
removed by mesmerism.

Unhappily, after being well nearly three years, she was

---

*Reich pointed out that in using an orgone energy accumulator, the
patient's biological energy must first be raised sufficiently to interact with
the energy of the accumulator, that orgonotically weak persons do not
feel any immediate effects. The same energetic situation apparently exists
between the physician-magnetiser and his patient.

terrified a third time on the 14th of June and suffered another relapse, and her mother came to me for assistance.

When I saw the girl she was feeble, almost sleepless, fearfully outrageous, having been sullen for the first three days. I easily sent her—who had been so long nearly sleepless—into a sleep which lasted from four that afternoon til ten the next morning. I desired the mother to continue to make the passes. Nothing else was done. The bowels soon became regular, and I saw the girl on Friday last, December 11, stout and in perfect health.

Some pertinent comments: It will be observed that when this patient was asleep, we left her. I have stated previously that if I had my own way, and had no reason from deviating from a general rule, *I would never wake a patient*. The longer the sleep the greater generally the benefit. Still, patients in their sleep-waking sometimes tell us that they should sleep only a certain time, and then we ought always—where there is no delirium—to follow their direction. Without such instructions, we may discover that sleep beyond a certain time does not leave them so well. This is, however, very seldom the case. Sometimes they grow uneasy in their sleep, and it is well to wake them and generally to send them to sleep again. But if none of these things take place I should never wish to wake a patient, nor do I except for mere convenience, as when they come to my house and I am obliged to go out at a certain hour, or when their avocations will not allow them to sleep beyond a certain time. They are sure to wake spontaneously sooner or later, as sure as we are from common sleep when we go to bed. Unfounded fear prevails that persons may never wake again from the mesmeric sleep, because it has appeared in the papers that persons could not be awakened. We sometimes wake them just when we wish, *but if we wait they will awake of their own accord*.

Case 18: Tic Douloureux*

Mr. H. U. Janson communicated this case which he treated with mesmerism. The case involves a Mrs. Canterbury of 48 Holloway Street. Mr. Janson's communication follows:

Mrs. Canterbury had been a martyr to the tic for four years before I knew her, during which time she took the advice of several physicians and surgeons in Exeter, but without any permanent benefit, though, as she told me, "The medicine sometimes seemed to have the effect of stunning the pain for the time, but it always returned with redoubled violence, so that no advantage was derived." The patient expressed her belief that the disease has been forming for a full eighteen years. It was therefore a thoroughly deep-rooted case.

Neuralgia, I may observe, appears to be one of the most mystic, or least explicable of all diseases. I do not require to be told that it is owing to a derangement of the nervous system, et cetera—that, of course, is admitted. But the question is, What causes this derangement?

One of my medical friends tells me it may be caused by disorder of almost any of the internal organs. As far as my own observation has gone, I am satisfied that these deep-rooted cases are frequently caused by the accumulation of a mass of matter in the chest. That it is so in this case I have not the slightest doubt, both from the self-evident symptoms of the case and also from the assertions of the patient herself during the trance.

---

*Tic is defined as a spasmodic muscular contraction, most commonly involving the face, head and neck. Tic douloureux is a degeneration of the trigeminal nerve resulting in neuralgia of that nerve.

The application of the mesmeric influence always produces a severe cough, which, by continuing the passes with energy, may be worked up so as to terminate in violent vomiting. In this way the amount of matter which has been removed is beyond calculation, for I have attended her now upwards of 300 times, and the process has been going on, more or less, from the commencement—though the expectoration began to diminish with the pain, and she has now for some time nearly ceased altogether. I have never heard of a worse case than this.

When I first became acquainted with Mrs. Canterbury she was, I verily believe, on the point of being starved to death, as the difficulty of eating a morsel of food was almost insurmountable. She told me that even to see preparations made for dinner was just the same to her as seeing a dentist preparing his instruments to drill her teeth. The least attempt at mastication would bring on such a paroxysm of agony that I have repeatedly seen the couch on which she lay tremble beneath her.

The skin of the face around the mouth peeled off, as it does from a patient after a fever. And both eating and speaking were becoming every day more and more impracticable. She used to receive me in perfect silence, lying on the sofa and merely pointing to a slate on which she had written any remarks she might have wished to make. In this state she would prepare for the operation (of mesmerism), looking the very picture of misery unutterable.

A very few minutes sufficed to place her in the mesmeric sleep, and anyone who entered an hour or so afterwards might indeed have stood astonished. There was my unutterably miserable patient sitting up, chatting, laughing, eating her dinner—not gruel and slops, but such things as steak and mutton chops—and looking as happy as possible. She would occasionally exclaim: "I cannot think how this is! I know I could not do this if you were not here!" For it is one of the peculiarities of this case that the patient has never, from the first, been in the slightest degree conscious of being in any other than her natural state, though she has not the slightest recollection after of anything that has occurred during the trance.

Many of my friends have come to see Mrs. Canterbury eat her dinner without her knowing it, and it really was quite a sight. I shall never forget the first time this experiment was tried. On being roused the patient looked much surprised and said, "Have I been eating?" I replied, "What makes you think so?" She said, "I have no recollection whatever of it, but I feel as if I had been dining sumptuously." "And well you may," said I, "for you have eaten a couple of mutton chops, a large piece of bread, and a considerable portion of pudding."

The astonishment depicted on my patient's face was most amusing. In this way she was gradually brought forward from weakness to strength. As soon as the violent coughing and expectoration—which usually took place as soon as the eyes were mesmerically closed—was quite over, I commenced the administration of edibles. This was done until at length the disease became so far subdued that my patient informed me she could eat comfortably awake.

I never heard of a more steady cure. The disease melted away, as Burns says, "Like snow wreaths in thaw." The dreadful paroxysms gradually died down to a few occasional twitches, which gradually diminished in number and severity, til she informed me that she had got over an entire day without the least pain. After that the improvement was rapid. She gained flesh and spirits and has now passed a full half a year without a single twitch or dart.

I think there is a point in our science which has not yet received sufficient attention—that is, I doubt whether a change in operators is beneficial to a patient. I have known several cases wherein a change of operators proved dreadfully injurious, and it appears to overthrow the benefit which had previously been effected. Lastly, I can truly say that I have never applied mesmerism continuously without producing decided benefit, if not a cure. Though in every one of them the ordinary remedies had proved "most superlatively useless." In fact it is, I think, the greatest thing in favor of mesmerism that nearly all our marvelous cures have been effected *after the Doctor has done all he can!*

I will conclude with this memorandum. As a copy of *The Zoist* is preserved in The British Museum, I wish to record for the astonishment of the men in 1946, that though the splendid case of Mrs. Canterbury has been a town's talk for nearly two years, yet during all that time *not a single medical practitioner who formerly attended her has ever once thought it worthwhile to request me to show or explain the case, or to ask me a single question about it!*

(signed) Henry Umpherville Janson
Pennsylvania Park, Exeter
August 18, 1846

Case 19: Palsy and Dropsy

The case of Martha Price, submitted by Mr. Decimus Hands, presents some unusual phenomena in a patient undergoing the mesmeric treatment. As we shall see, the patient herself began to actively participate in the direction of her treatment. She did this during her somnambulistic state, or while she was in sleep-waking. Although the entire case is somewhat lengthy, it provides enough worthwhile material to be examined with care.

May 24, 1844: Martha Price is nineteen years of age, short, thick set, dark hair and eyes. She has been suffering from dropsy of the abdomen, chest, and whole body—with trembling in the limbs and throughout the muscles generally. She is subject to morning perspirations, giddiness, taste and smell impaired—especially the former. She complains of palpitation of the heart, with a sense of its being tied down and not having room to act. Catamenia scanty. Motion produces pain in the limbs, even in the fingers. She also suffers constipation, sleepless nights, and palsy of the left arm and leg.

This day I commenced mesmerizing Martha Price by making long passes downwards very slowly from the top of the head. I continued for about three-quarters of an hour without producing any apparent result, all of which time she laughed immoderately. Then her eyes assumed the heavy appearance peculiar to the mesmeric state and soon closed so that she could not open them when, as it was late, I demesmerized her and she returned home and slept better than she had done since her illness.

The next day she was again mesmerized with apparently no better success. But on her return home, while at dinner she fell asleep—in the strict meaning of the words—for the knife and fork dropped from her hands, so suddenly did she lose consciousness. She was put to bed and slept from 1 to 6 P.M., and again at night from midnight til 8 A.M.

May 26: Mesmerized as usual. Nothing occurred worthy of remark; yet there was a decided improvement, for she could lie down, which she had not been able to do since her breathing had been so bad. The pain, however, was still acute and the appetite nearly failed.

May 27: This day for the first time Martha went into the mesmeric sleep, though only for a very short interval.

May 28: She again slept and complained of pain in the stomach. From this day her loss of consciousness gradually increased in duration, and her breathing ameliorated in proportion to the length of the sleep. The stomach and chest, which were swollen, decreased in size. Before she was mesmerized the kidneys had become nearly inactive. After the third day of mesmerization, they had resumed their functions, so that there was frequent and long-continued micturation. This I concluded to have been the result of the absorbance having been stimulated into activity by the magnetic influence, thus draining off the contents of the cavities and cellular membrane generally. In the course of twelve hours the patient passed six pints of water.

May 29: Catamenia came on a fortnight before the right period—they had been regular hitherto.

May 30: During the sleep I perceived a slight spasm in the right arm.

May 31: This day the spasm became more decided. *In her sleep she now began to direct my operations.* She desired me to make longitudinal passes, commencing at the top of her head and going very slowly down the left side of the head, face, neck, and shoulder to the end of the fingers. As I proceeded I observed *red streaks rising from under my fingers,* resembling inflamed absorbance. I continued these passes til the whole surface bore the appearance of a person who had been the subject *of ardent scarlet fever!*

The passes over the head produced excruciating pain in the face, eye, and limbs of the left side, and lastly in the head, heart, and side. The agony was so intense as to contort all her features, causing her to grind her teeth and move her jaws convulsively. She described the pain as the sensation of the blood flowing to the head and boiling and bubbling in the brain. The arm and hand—with the leg and foot of the same side—were stretched out and elongated, raised up and lowered by *my passes and will combined.* The passes made from above downwards, along the extensor muscles, excited the flexors into action. And if I made passes in the same direction along the flexors, then a similar effect was produced in the extensors.

This same day I placed gold in her hand, when the fingers closed immediately, though slowly upon it, forming a fist. The wrist joint flexed upwards, the elbow in like manner toward the shoulder. The whole of the flexor muscles of the superior extremity being evidently influenced by the gold and with a violence sufficient to have crushed to atoms a glass smelling-bottle she had in her hand, had I not hastily wrested it from her before the full development of the mesmeric influence of the muscles.

I had ceased de-mesmerizing her for some days, as she always awoke when I left the room. The following is taken down from her dictation:

> On the 31st of May, after Mr. Hands left me, I awoke as usual and on rising from my chair I felt three distinct cracks in my side, shooting down to my leg and foot, which made me scream out each time. It was like a knife running through me, and just the same pain I felt when first seized on the 14th of February. I then found I could move my leg and arm, and that feeling had returned to my side. I thought I would try and walk home, as it was not a great distance, and accordingly I did walk from 18 Upper York Street to Johns Street New Road where I lived, holding by the iron railing of the areas. I passed my mother and sister as they were coming to fetch me. I turned away my head and they did not see me, for I wished to enjoy their amazement. The next day I determined to astonish Mr. Hands, and walked to his house, 22 Thayer Street.

Indeed, it would be difficult to imagine the delighted surprise with which I received such an encouraging proof of the curative power of mesmerism. The exertion did not prove in the least prejudicial to Martha. The same phenomena were again elicited with increased strength. She conceived that "a string which had contracted the limb snapped in two," and now the leg was at liberty. She complained of weakness in the back of the neck and head. The bowels were confined; the kidneys again being partially inactive. The sleep continued good. Nothing worthy of note occurred for several days. Laughing always awoke her.

On one occasion my friend, the Reverend Mr. Bridgeman, had been amusing her in relating some entertaining stories, and consequently continually awaking her, when the question crossed his mind whether his *thinking* of anything droll would have the same effect. He immediately put the idea into action, and to his great surprise she awoke as quickly and quite as much amused as if he had given utterance to the thought. However, I had only to hold up my hand—and though she might not see me, she would go to sleep instantly.

June 14: She was suffering from headache brought on by exposure to cold. I merely touched her fingers and she went into the sleep.

June 26: I asked her in her sleep when she would be well of the paralysis. She considered for some time and replied, "In three weeks."

July 2: I sat down at the distance of three feet from Martha and merely looked at her. She fell asleep in four minutes. For the first time, she leaned towards me. I moved around her chair and she followed my movements, leaning over to me as much as she possibly could without falling. I then sat down and immediately stood up again, when she made two ineffectual attempts at imitation, but the third time succeeded, stood up erect and sat down directly. Someone present laughed, and she awoke and was surprised at what we told her she had done.

July 9: She now asserted in her sleep she would be quite well in a week. The fulfillment of this prediction is proved by the fact that she went to a situation as housemaid to a lady residing in Oxford Street on the 22nd of July.

MARTHA'S RELAPSE

On Monday, July 22, Martha went to her place (of employment) exactly eight weeks from the time she had first been mesmerized. On the subsequent Friday, as she was shaking up a bed, she felt a sensation pass through her side like a flash of lightning. It darted upwards to the eye, which closed. She recognized the pain and hastily slid down the stairs holding the baluster, and succeeded in reaching the bottom before her foot and leg were seized. This attack was much more aggravated than the former. The left eye remained shut, and the entire side was paralyzed.

During her stay at home she had gone through a severe mental trial, which doubtless had contributed to predispose her to this relapse. She first felt numbness in her leg and arm, then in the fingers and up the course of the radial nerve. Next, the extremities of the left side were quite paralyzed. The pulse was slow and soft. She had night perspirations. Just prior to the attack she experienced a sense of vacancy in the stomach and had a severe fit of sneezing.

I was sent for and mesmerized her immediately. But though she went into the sleep, she derived no apparent benefit. The next day she directed me to draw off the vesical contents with an instrument while she was asleep—the vesica being paralyzed, which I did, but it soon accumulated again. She assured me the water came from the legs, being—as I had before concluded—absorbed and conveyed through the ordinary channels to the vesica.

She was removed home that evening, when I again mesmerized her. Gold, which had acted so powerfully in her previous illness, now failed in producing any effect. On the Sunday while she was asleep, the closed eye rolled slowly open, presenting the frightful object of a sightless orb. After a short time it reclosed. But when she woke it opened naturally like the other, and she found she had recovered the use of it.

July 29: In her sleep she desired me to take sixteen ounces of blood. . . . Now there was an exact repetition of all the former violent contortions of the 31st of May, but with increasing power. There was the closing of the fingers, the flexing of the wrist and elbow joints—but now, after the latter had folded upwards toward the shoulder, it slowly lowered itself and kept stretching out with convulsive jerks: the flexor muscles slowly contracting and the extensors darting forwards until the power of both sets of muscles had regained ability to perform their functions and the arm was fully elongated.

July 30: In her sleep she said she must be kept very quiet and drink barley water and eat a small amount of bread, that she must be bled again on the next Monday, after which she would have the use of her limbs. She assured me mesmerism would cure her, and told me to draw off the vesical content before I made passes over the legs. She fancied that *she saw letters on her heart,* but confusedly—she said she should see them better another day.

July 31: In her sleep she said she felt something very hot pass through her, hot, like steam from my forehead. My fingers gave her pain. She saw fluid passing up and down her heart. The "letters" now appeared clear, some upside down. She fancied the word "salivation" and "mercury," but immediately corrected herself and said that the latter word was "a guess. But I see twelve small pills of bluish color. I must take them and they will produce salivation and operate on the bowels," which had been confined for several days.

Aug 2: While "reading the letters upon her heart," Martha's appearance was most singular. She appeared to be looking down and searching about, peering into the interior recesses of her heart. She compared herself to "a hen with a brood under her wing." At times she appeared perplexed, then would brighten up and her countenance sparkle with pleasure. She described the letters as if "written with a fiery pencil, *and all light*." She likewise searched into the head and brain—the left side of which she saw covered with blood. (While she was in the hospital, every application was directed toward the right side.) She had begun her pills, taking one twice a day.

August 3: Her bowels acted as she had prognosticated. She slept three-quarters of an hour and said her mouth would be affected when she had taken four more pills. She directed me to draw off the vesical content, but not to put gold in her hand for it drew the blood from her head; I must therefore use it when I bleed her.

Aug. 5: The bowels acted, and micturation occurred twice.

August 6: I took away more blood. The catamenia came on. She said that when they ceased she would be quite well. *She, now in her sleep, always "read on her heart" and directed me what to do.* Sensibility was recovered in four toes; the middle one remained insensible. Salivation began; the pills were finished.

August 7: She was very red. While in the mesmeric sleep she assured me she would be quite well when she awoke— meaning that she would have regained sensation and feeling in all her limbs and no longer suffer from paralysis. She was not able to leave her bed yet, as she was too weak, and there was still the dropsy, which would not yield quite so soon, but with perseverance she should be cured of that in a little time.

I placed my hand on the top of her head, which had been hitherto so painful to the touch. She fancied there was a string covered with bloody knots that tied it. I produced pain and spasm of the right arm and leg. I put a mesmerized sovereign on her shoulder and she fancied the string broke. Her head had been drawn over her shoulder, and when I removed the sovereign the head fell back to its place.

As I passed my hand over the head, tears flowed copiously down the cheeks, especially from the eye that had been affected. The back of her head felt "dead," and she said she could not bear the couch to touch one part of it. She said it felt as if a piece of the brain was loose and fell against the forehead when she leaned forwards. *She fancied matter was forming on the brain like a scab which would soon appear outwardly on the skin in the shape of scales* and would have to be brushed off. The itching sensation was terrible, and was relieved by grinding the teeth and shaking the head which seemed "to scratch it."

Martha said my being in the room was sufficient of itself to send her to sleep. She said that there was a large collection of water in the abdomen in a sac, but more on the right side than on the left.

The following Monday, catamenia came on. She said they would continue until Wednesday. She must not take medicine, for mesmerized water would produce the same effect. A few days later Martha said the water in the peritoneum had been so agitated by the magnetic power that it was now nearly gone. She wished to have her head shaved, and we had the demonstration of the truth of her prediction: *There was a large oval place about the size and shape of a section of an egg, having the appearance of dandruff and of a darkish color.*

About this time Martha's mother was confined, and as she required her daughter's services, we were obliged to discontinue mesmerism for rather more than a fortnight, after which period we again resumed. But Martha said the interval had been pernicious—the peritoneum having again filled, and that it would require twenty-four hours of uninterrupted sleep for the water to be absorbed and carried off. We therefore settled that she should come the next day, Saturday, to her friend's house, and that I should send her to sleep at eleven o'clock, which I did. But she had not been asleep long before she became restless and appeared uncomfortable. She had not acquainted her mother with her intention, and she said she saw her mother very angry.

I offered to go to her mother and get someone to do the work instead of Martha. To this she consented and on my return I told her her mother was quite satisfied. But I had hardly left the house before Martha peremptorily ordered her friend to awaken her, who very naturally refused and remonstrated with her, telling her that I should be most justly offended after the trouble I had taken, especially as her mother had offered no objection. Martha then asked for two bunches of keys and her wedding ring; and as there was but one bunch of keys, she took off the largest key, placed it in one hand, the bunch in the other, the ring on her forehead, *and instantly awoke!*

But now arose a fresh difficulty—she refused to go home! Nothing could be more striking than the contrast presented between Martha in the mesmeric sleep and Martha awake: whereas in the one she was all nervous, anxious, and solicitous of appeasing and conciliating her mother, in the other she was as tenacious and obstinate not to concede in the least to what she deemed her mother's ill temper.

However, at length she returned home, but when her mother saw her she was frightened at her appearance and sent her back immediately. She passed a very bad night, and when I saw her on Sunday I was much surprised at all that had happened.

I sent her to sleep immediately, and she said that all the alteration had been very pernicious, and that in consequence

it would be necessary now that she should sleep three nights
and three days without waking. I must de-mesmerize her
that evening, and then send her to sleep again and leave her
undisturbed til the following Wednesday. In the evening I
awoke her as she desired. She took some refreshment and I
sent her to sleep again. She told us she should talk and eat
on Monday and Tuesday, but would be too ill on the Wednesday and continue insensible all the day til her waking
hour—six o'clock in the evening, when we should find the
dropsy quite gone.

During the sleep, she was seen by many persons, including Dr. Elliotson, the Reverend G. Sandby, and Mr. Atkinson. *As soon as Dr. Elliotson entered the room, she named
him, though she had never seen him!* And when asked how
she knew him and not the others, she said he was "one of
the family," and explained that each person I had mesmerized was "lit up by the mesmeric fluid" and she read their
names.

I now hasten to the Wednesday evening, half an hour
before the appointed time for her awaking. Her breathing
was curious—she had lain all day apparently unconscious
with imperceptible breathing. Now it became deep—very
deep—then again it nearly ceased. At times there was a restless moaning and the frame energetically contorted, relapsing
afterwards into apparent insensibility. The Reverend G.
Sandby and Mr. Atkinson were present. Dr. Elliotson was
prevented by an engagement. We were all anxiously awaiting
with our watches in our hands when the church clock opposite struck, and Martha was awake in an instant.

I was fearful she might be agitated on seeing the two
gentlemen who were strangers to her, but she was quite calm,
as I remained near. The next day when I called I found her
very weak, and on sending her to sleep she complained of
cold and of suffering from the looseness of the integuments

of the abdomen. The water having been all absorbed and carried off, she directed me to apply a bandage eight yards long.

Before I arrived she had prevailed on a friend to give her a quantity of very hot potatoes, which she ate greedily. She said she suffered so very much from internal cold and they warmed her.

From this day her recovery may be considered complete, for she had no return of any of the symptoms, either of dropsy or of paralysis, but continued to gain strength daily. Her clairvoyance increased likewise—and she soon was equally clever in discerning and in prescribing for diseases in others as she had done for herself. I have only to state further that at the present time, though not a strong woman, she is perfectly able to undertake any light situation in a private family, and that it is now nearly two years since her recovery, which I date from the last sleep—September 1844.

(signed) Decimus Hands
24 August, 1846

Case 20: Cancer of the Breast

This case of cancer of the breast is presented by Dr. Elliotson. Treatment by Animal Magnetism spanned a period of five years. The case, as we shall see, was diagnosed by several physicians, and radical surgery was suggested by most.

On March 6, 1843, a very respectable looking person of middle age and height, fair, rather slender and delicate, and with the sallow complexion of cancer, called to solicit my advice respecting a disease of her right breast. I found an intensely hard tumor in the center of the breast—circumscribed, movable, and apparently five or six inches in circumference. The part was drawn in and puckered, as though a string attached behind the skin at one point had pulled the surface inwards; and upon it, to the outer side of the nipple, was a dry, rough, warty-looking substance of a dirty brown and greenish color.

She complained of great tenderness in the tumor and the armpit when I applied my fingers, and said that she had sharp stabbing pains through the tumor during the day and was continually awakened by them during the night.

The woman was single. Upon minute inquiry into the origin, course, and duration of the complaint, I found that one day in November 1841, while sitting at rest after having finished some dresses (she was a seamstress), she raised her right hand to take something off the mantle and instantly felt a sudden and violent darting pain in the right breast. In a week, she felt a second, equally violent. These "dreadful dartings," to use her own words, soon ceased to be solitary and began at length to take place a dozen times in rapid succession every few hours. The dartings were always followed by pricking sensations and tenderness.

Her complexion and hands had gradually grown sallow for months. She mentioned her complaint about six months ago, before I saw her, to a medical man, Mr. Powell of Brunswick Square, while he was attending her brother, but declined showing it to him as he was a young man.

Her father's mother had died of bleeding cancer of the breast. As she had witnessed a mesmeric cure of a niece, I proposed mesmerism to her and offered to take the charge of the case myself. *My purpose was to render her insensible to the surgical removal of the breast,* seeing no other chance for her, and this indeed was a poor chance, for cancer invariably returns to the same or some part if the patient survives long enough. And the operation is not to be recommended unless it can be conducted without pain. When a disease termed "cancer" has not returned, I have no doubt that it has not been cancer. And such a terrible thing as the removal of breasts not cancerous has always been too frequent among surgeons.

Unwilling to make her unhappy, I said no more and allowed her to suppose that the mesmerism was intended to cure her illness. She accepted my offer and returned to my house the next day for the first attempt.

I mesmerised her half an hour daily with slow passes before her, from opposite her forehead to opposite her stomach, and my fixed look at her eyes. The first mesmerisation caused a mistiness before her eyes at the time and a much better night than usual. In a few days she became a bit drowsy, and at the end of a month her eyes perfectly closed and she fell asleep near the expiration of the half hour. The sleep however was slight and a word to her, or the least touch of my fingers, awoke her. I could not distinguish it from natural sleep. *There was no increase of effect for nine months.** She seldom slept much longer than half an hour, frequently much less, though a dozen passes were sufficient to send her back into sleep.

The pain lessened so that her nights became greatly better, and her health and spirits improved. The sallowness of her complexion lessened. But for six months she continued to work hard making dresses, so that she once fainted at Hampstead. Also, *for the first six months of mesmerisation the tumor increased,* though every other symtom improved. The act of pushing a needle through hard articles gave her pain to the very elbow. Finally she could work no longer and in September lost the whole of her business.

A niece, whom she had taken to benevolently support eleven years before—when the girl's mother was unexpectedly left with nine children—having learnt that her

---

*A less dedicated physician might easily have given up the process long ago. As will be shown, however, great perseverance paid off.

aunt's disease was cancer, suddenly left her without any explanation or apology. It afterwards transpired that the girl said she would not nurse her aunt through her illness, which she of course concluded would be tedious and fatal.

I had felt it right to mention the nature of the disease to her niece's mother, and all the family thus knew it but kept it secret. A fortnight after she first came to see me, one of the ladies who employed her begged that she would see Mr. Brown, practicing in Edgeware Road. The patient consented without my knowledge. Mr. Brown pronounced it to be no cancer but a common glandular swelling from a strain, and he wished to send her a plaster. However, he saw it again in September, again without my knowledge, and had no doubt that it was cancer. This candid acknowledgement was highly creditable to him, no less than his remark respecting mesmerism. He spoke against the surgical operation, adding that if the patient were his sister she should not submit to one; and not being able to suggest a remedy he made no attempt to dissuade her from the influence of mesmerism, but said that he knew nothing about it and therefore should say nothing against it. This display of common sense is deserving of all imitation by medical men.

Soon after Mr. Brown had seen it the first time, she showed it at her mother's request to Mr. Powell, who immediately in her presence pronounced it to be a confirmed "incurable cancer," adding that if it were not "cut away it would be as big as a head by Christmas," and that if mesmerism cured it, he would believe anything. She thus learnt the distressing truth which I had so anxiously kept from her.

The various ladies felt so much for her that they anxiously urged her to undergo the operation, some begging and praying, and some most kindly offering to nurse her and sit up with her after the operation. One, a relation of Sir

Benjamin Brodie, was hurt with her because she would not place herself under Sir Benjamin's care. Like a true-hearted woman, she resisted all these well-intentioned influences behind my back and remained firm to him in whom she had placed her confidence.

In September I left England for a tour of the Pyrenees til November, and left her to be mesmerised daily by a gentleman whom I allowed 200 pounds per annum, with a constant place at my table, to mesmerise for me gratuitously and investigate the subject with me.

During the early part of my absence, Mr. Powell saw the patient again and anxiously urged immediate removal with the knife. He mentioned Sir Benjamin Brodie and Mr. Liston, but she declined. He then entreated her to accompany him to Mr. Samuel Cooper, Professor of Surgery at University College, who he was sure would see her without a fee, and at length she consented. Mr. Cooper differed from Mr. Powell in thinking that the operation could not be safely delayed til my return, but he gave a decided opinion that the disease was cancer and that the operation should be performed as soon as ever I came back. "Poor thing," said this good and kind man. "If she wishes to wait for Dr. Elliotson's return, she may, but it must be cut away then."

On my return I found she had not been mesmerised to the extent I wished, and was therefore not so susceptible as when I left her. But I took her in hand again myself, and in less than two months she passed into genuine sleep-waking, with perfect insensibility to mechanical injury. Mr. Powell called upon her two or three times, wishing to see the breast and try once to mesmerise her, but she declined and he ceased to call upon her, nor did he ever communicate with me upon the subject of her case.

Her health continued to improve, the pains to lessen, and the size was stationary. In February, failing to appear

at my house, I went to see her at her mother's lodgings in
Nutford Place, Brianstone Square. She was laboring under
severe pleurisy of the right side and required bleeding.
Without her knowing it, she was bled, at my request, by
Mr. Ebbsworth.

The venousection had been followed by a bruised appearance of the arm. I advised her friend to rub the arm
downward, which was done in her sleep, and rigidity of
the limb took place. Any part of her could, from this time,
be made rigid. She was soon able to repeat her daily visits
to my house. I recommended that her mother or a little
orphan niece who lived with them should also mesmerise
her morning and evening, and that they should in her sleep-
waking make contact passes upon her breast over the linen.
I did this myself over her dress at every opportunity.

She was so susceptible that not merely a single pass but
a look always caused her upper eyelids to quiver and descend
and close and sleep-waking to come on. She was always
perfectly relaxed and powerless in every part, and always
perfectly insensible from head to foot to mechanical causes
of pain. Yet she felt contact, or resistance and temperature,
whether hot or cold. I recollect the incredulous look which
these phenomena of feeling excited in various persons when
I exhibited them. But ether and chloroform have produced
the same phenomena, and not a single medical man has,
in a single instance, expressed a single doubt upon *their*
reality when produced by these narcotic drugs!

It is a common thing for mesmerised patients to be insensible to pinching, cutting, pricking, and tearing—and yet
to be perfectly sensible of the temperature of cold and
warm substances applied to the very same parts, and to be
sensible if they are touched or pressed.

Hundreds have been astonished at the patient's rigidity.
By firm contact passes down her arms as she lay in an easy

chair, I stiffened them; then her legs, then her whole trunk, so that her body could not be bent; then her neck so that her head could not be bent, then her jaw so that she could not speak; then her lips so that she could not move them in the least.

This rigidity would last for hours. And though the sleep-waking now continued much longer than before—perhaps for hours—it sometimes ceased, while the rigidity continued. Sometimes the rigidity ceased before the sleep-waking. This state of rigidity deepened and lengthened the sleep, as it generally does, and strengthened her. As a general rule, not only ought patients be allowed to continue in the sleep-waking til this terminates spontaneously, but they should be stiffened and allowed to remain so for the purpose of greater invigoration. If relaxation comes on, they should be stiffened again.

When patients have been fairly sent into sleep-waking, so that contact and moving do not waken them, firm longitudinal contact passes should be regularly made upon their limbs as long as possible in the hope of at length inducing the phenomenon of rigidity.

Soon this rigidity could be induced in any part by the same means *in her waking state*. And the part always became at the same time insensible, as in her sleep-waking. Whether awake or asleep she could be molded into any form, by putting her limbs, the head or the body in the desired position and then stiffening the parts. Or her jaw only could be locked, so that if awake she could look and walk, but not talk.

If many parts were stiffened in her waking state, sleep soon overpowered her and lasted long, and the rigidity still continued. If a relaxed arm was bent upwards toward the shoulder, and contact passes made inside it, as if to draw it toward the shoulder, it would grow rigid thus, bent upon the shoulder. No ordinary force could draw it down. Pulling on the arm pulled the whole body forward, but the arm did not move one-half inch from the body. Yet, by contact passes, ever so gentle upon the arm, as though you wished to bring the arm down, it presently loosened and then fell perfectly relaxed in her lap. In some patients, the part drawn does not relax, but rigidly assumes the new position to which you bring it.

Any part of this patient could be readily relaxed by breathing upon it, by touching it with even the point of a finger or with an inanimate substance, by perfectly transverse passes across it, by darting the hand at it, or by contact passes in the opposite direction to that in which the part was contracted.

The summer of 1844 passed on. The cancerous sallowness disappeared. She had less pain, her strength increased, and the warty-looking growth dropped off, leaving a sound, smooth surface, and there was no increase of the diseased substance. Dr. Ashburner saw the part, had no hesitation of calling the disease cancer, and was delighted at the favorable prospect. A surgical operation was therefore not thought of.

[Despite some setbacks in the progress of this case, Dr. Elliotson continued with his treatment through the summer of 1845 and then 1846, when, near the end of August, she had another attack of pleurisy accompanied by bronchitis, from which she recovered.]

The present year, 1848, arrived. She has had catarrh and a fit of asthma several times. The fit of asthma was always removed by my laying my hands upon her chest over her clothes for ten minutes in her mesmeric state. The tumor continued to decrease and the tenderness to wear off, and the gland in the armpit disappeared.

The cancerous mass is now completely dissipated. The

breast is perfectly flat, and all the skin rather thicker and firmer than before the disease existed. Not the slightest lump is to be found, nor is there the slightest tenderness of the bosom or the armpit.

Case 21: Removal of a Breast

The ability of mesmerism to render patients insensitive to pain has been shown in the many cases already presented. Once the pain-deadening qualities of this method were established, its use as a general anesthetic in major and minor surgery was merely a logical extension of its application in non-surgical cases.

The following authentic cases are only a brief sampling of the hundreds of other surgical procedures performed in the middle and late nineteenth century, in which mesmerism was the sole agent used to anesthetize the patient. They appear here, for the most part, in their original historical presentation with only minor changes made for the sake of clarity.

Dr. L. A. Ducas, Professor of Physiology in the Medical College of Georgia (U.S.A.), wrote up this case for the *Southern Medical and Surgical Journal*, after performing the operation in the presence of several eminent physicians.

On the third of January, 1845, Mrs. Clark, wife of Mr. Jess Clark of Columbia County, Georgia, came to the city for the purpose of getting me to remove a scirrhous tumor of the right breast, which had been gradually increasing for the last three years and had now attained the size of a turkey's egg. The tumor had never caused any pain of consequence, was not adhering to the skin, nor did it implicate any of the axillary glands.

Mrs. Clark is about forty-seven years of age, has never

borne a child, and her health—by no means robust—was pretty good and had not been impaired by the evolution of the tumor.

The operation having been determined upon for the following day, Mrs. Clark remarked to me that she had been advised by Mr. Kendrick to be mesmerised. But as she knew nothing about mesmerism she would ask my advice and abide by it. To which I replied that there were several well-authenticated cases on record in which surgical operations had been performed under mesmeric influence without the consciousness of the patient. I told her I would be happy to test mesmerism in her case, and that I would endeavor to mesmerise her instead of operating, as had been proposed, on the following day.

On January 4th, at 11 A.M., I called on Mrs. Clark and was informed that, on the preceding evening, she had been put to sleep by Mr. B. F. Kendrick, at whose house she resided. I then mesmerised her myself and induced sleep in about fifteen minutes. Finding my patient susceptible to the mesmeric influence, and reflecting that it would not be convenient for the same person to maintain this influence and to perform the surgical operation at the same time, I requested Mr. Kendrick to mesmerise Mrs. Clark morning and evening, at stated hours, until insensibility could be induced. This was regularly done with gradually increasing effect, when, on the evening of the 6th January, sleep was induced in five minutes and the prick of a pin was attended with no manifestation of pain.

The sittings were continued and the patient's insensibility daily tested by myself and others in various ways. On January 9th I invited Professor Ford to be present, and after pricking and pinching strongly, and the patient evidencing no pain, we exposed the breast, handled it roughly in examining the tumor, and readjusted the dress without the patient being conscious of it. We then held to her nostrils a vial of strong spirits of hartshorn, which she breathed freely for a minute or so without the least indication of sensation.

On January 11th, in the presence of Professors Ford and Mead, in addition to the usual tests, I made with my pocket knife an incision about two inches in length and a half-inch in depth into the patient's leg without indication of sensation. Fully satisfied now of our power to induce total insensibility, I determined to operate on her the next day at noon, but carefully concealed any such design from the patient and her friends, who did not expect its performance until several days later.

On January 12th, at twenty minutes past 11 A.M., Mrs. Clark was put to sleep in forty-five seconds. At twelve o'clock noon, in the presence of Professors Ford, Mead, Garvin, Newton, and Dr. Halsey, the patient being in a profound sleep, I prepared her dress for the operation and requested my professional brothers to note her pulse, respiration, complexion, countenance, et cetera, before, during, and after the amputation, in order to detect any evidence of pain or modification of the functions.

As Mr. Kendrick had never witnessed a surgical operation, he feared he might lose his self-possession and requested that he be blindfolded, which was done. He now seated himself on the couch near the patient and held her hand in his during the operation. The operation was accomplished by two elliptical incisions about eight inches in length, comprehending between them the nipple and a considerable portion of the skin, after which the integuments were dissected up in the usual manner and the entire breast removed. It weighed 16 ounces.

The wound was then left open about three-quarters of an hour in order to secure the bleeding vessels, six of which were ligated. The ordinary dressing was applied and all appearances of blood carefully removed so that they might not be seen by the patient when aroused. The amount of hemorrhage was rather more than usual in such cases.

During the operation the patient gave no indication whatsoever of sensibility, nor were any of the functions observed to those present modified in the least degree. She remained in the same quiet sleep as before the use of the knife. Subsequently, the pectoral muscle, which had been laid bare, was twice or thrice seen to contract when touched with a sponge in removing blood.

Fifteen minutes after the operation, a tremulous action was perceived in the lower jaw, which was instantaneously arrested by the application of the mesmeriser's hand to the patient's head. This phenomenon recurred in about ten minutes after, and was again in the same manner requited.

Professor Ford, who counted the pulse and respiration, states that before any preparation was made for the operation the pulse was 96 and the respiration 16 per minute. And after removing the patient to arrange her dress for the operation, her pulse was 98 and respiration 17. Immediately after the detachment of the breast, the pulse was 96, respiration not counted. And after the final adjustment of the bandages and dress, which required the patient to rise and move about, the pulse was 98 and the respiration 16.

All present concur in stating that neither the placid countenance of the patient nor the peculiar natural blush of the cheeks experienced any change during the whole process, that she continued in the same profound and quiet sleep in which she was before noted, and that had they not been aware of what was being done they would not have suspected it from any indications furnished by the patient's condition.

The patient having been permitted to sleep on for about

a half an hour after the final arrangement of her dress, the mesmeriser made passes over the site of the operation in order to lessen its sensibilities and aroused her in the usual manner, at which time she engaged Mr. Kendrick and myself in cheerful conversation as though she had no suspicion of what had taken place.

After a few minutes of conversation I asked her when she would like to have the operation performed, to which she replied, "The sooner the better," as she was anxious to get home. I added, "Do you really think that I could remove your entire breast when asleep without your knowledge?"

Answer: "Why, Doctor, the fact is that from the various experiments I am told you have made on me, I really do not know what to think of it."

"Well, madam, suppose I were to perform the operation one of these days and to inform you of it when you would awake. Would you believe me? And could you control your feelings on finding that it had been done?"

Answer: "I could not suppose that you would deceive me, and of course I would be very glad, but would try not to give way to my feelings."

"Have you perceived, since your arrival here, or do you now perceive any change in the ordinary sensations of the affected breast?"

"No, sir. It feels about as it has done for some time back."

Thereupon I informed her that the breast had been removed. She said I was certainly jesting, as it was impossible that it could have been done without her knowing it at the time or feeling anything of it now. She became convinced only on carrying her hand to the part and finding that the breast was no longer there. She remained apparently unmoved for a few moments. When her friends approached to congratulate her, her face became flushed and she wept unaffectedly for some time. The wound healed by the first intention.*

Case 22: Removal of a Polypus from the Nose

The following case of surgery was performed by Albert T. Wheelock, M.D., and written up in the *Boston Medical and Surgical Journal*. Dr. Wheelock's account follows:

Additional to the accounts of like results that have lately reached us from various quarters, an experiment has dragged me into being a witness of the particulars that are hereby detailed to you as follows, for what they are worth, concerning the removal in July 1843 of a polypus from the nose of a patient in the mesmeric condition. I give this name ("mesmerism") to the condition she was in for want of a better one, but names are of little consequence, the facts only—from notes taken at the time—being intended to be regarded.

The patient came from Montville, fourteen miles distant, to Belfast for the purpose of having the operation. She was a very respectable woman of mild disposition and manners, of considerable energy and activity, fair complexion, about twenty-four years of age, married, had one child, was a person of good constitution, and to every appearance healthy at the time.

The tumor was an oblong, rounded form, largely attached base, probably half an inch in its smallest diameter, and had been there about three months. The base was larger proportionally than the average of cases within my experience and so firmly adherent that in removing it I was obliged to tear it away in pieces.

I had laid out my instruments and was about to proceed

---

*Without granulation or suppuration.

in the operation when the patient proposed to be magnetized, if it was possible, as she dreaded the pain that would
have to be borne.

As she was entirely unacquainted in town, at her request
I procured the attendance of a gentleman who had the
reputation of being a good magnetiser—Mr. Phineas T.
Quimby,* who consented to aid the woman. For my part,
I was entirely without faith in the procedure, as I told the
patient at that time, and as I had told others previously who
had asked me what I thought of Animal Magnetism. I am
quite confident that the lady and Mr. Quimby had never
met before and that there was nothing previously concerted.
I am also confident that she took no medicine to induce
stupor.

In ten minutes after commencing, she was put into a
state of apparently natural sleep, sitting upright in her chair
—breathing and pulse natural, color of countenance un-
changed. We then moved her from the back part of my
room, where she happened to be sitting, to a window for the
light.

Mr. Quimby asked her if she felt well. She said distinctly,
"Yes." I immediately, in the presence of several of our most
noted citizens, who had been called in at their own request,
began to remove the tumor, and did it thoroughly, scraping
the sides of the nostril repeatedly with a forceps so as to
be sure I had removed all the remaining fragments.

There was some hemorrhage, nearly an ounce of blood.
I was operating four or five minutes at least. During the
whole time she evinced not the slightest symptom of pain,

---

*This is the same Phineas Quimby who treated Mary Baker Eddy,
founder of the Christian Science Church. After being helped by the magnetiser, Mrs. Eddy nevertheless turned on her benefactor and denounced
Animal Magnetism with vehemence.

either by any groaning, sighing, or motion whatever, but was in all these respects exactly like the dead body.

I felt convinced that I might as well have amputated her arm. The circumstance that struck me at the time most singularly of all was this: As soon as the blood began to run down the throat, she made a slight rough, rattling sound of breathing. One of the bystanders said, "She is choking to death!" *Mr. Quimby then cleared his throat and spit repeatedly, and the lady did the same and spit the blood out of her mouth!*

About ten minutes after the operation she was awakened, but said she was unconscious that anything had been done. She complained of no pain, and found that she could now breathe freely through her nose that had been entirely closed up for several preceding months.

Case 23: Amputation of a Leg

This case of amputation of a leg occurred at Cherbourg, October 2, 1845.

Miss Mary Dollbanell, seventeen years of age, had labored for many years under a disease of the right foot occasioned by a sprain. For above three years amputation had been pronounced inevitable. But, not withstanding the progress of the disease, the patient could never be brought to consent to an operation which the most courageous man never contemplates without dread.

At length it was determined to have recourse to mesmerism in order to render her insensible to pain, and in order to perform the operation, the necessity for which was every day more imminent, without her knowledge.

She was mesmerised by Mr. Durand, who had no doubt of success, and the result proved the accuracy of his judgment. The first effect of mesmerism was the restoraion of Miss Dollbanell's appetite and sleep, of which she had been very long deprived. The degree of her insensibility, having been frequently examined, was at length found to be such as was necessary, and she consented during her sleep-waking to submit to the operation—or, rather, she earnestly entreated to have it performed.

The amputation was fixed for the following Thursday, October 2, at twelve-thirty. On the day fixed, at eleven o'clock, Miss Dollbanell was sent to sleep in less than three minutes and then placed upon a table. Preparations were immediately made in her presence, and as soon as Mr. Durand was satisfied that the insensibility was deep and positive, he informed the surgeons that they might begin the operation with perfect certainty.

Then, in the midst of a solemn silence—and while all the assistants were fixing an attentive and scrutinizing eye upon the peaceful countenance of the patient—Dr. Loysel made a large circular incision with his knife, which penetrated deeply into the flesh as far as the bone, and bared the greater part of the tibia and fibula. The blood flowed abundantly. The two flaps were cut and dissected, the periosteum cut, the bone sawn; the ligatures of the arteries, the cleansing and putting up of the wound, the application of the bandages and lint, all this was done without the patient giving the slightest symptom of pain.

Her countenance continued calm and undisturbed. Her hands remained constantly free, and she several times smiled and conversed with her mesmeriser, even during the most painful stages of the operation, which, including the putting up, lasted about half an hour.

The insensibility was complete. The patient had no knowledge of what was happening. The pulse underwent no change in either strength or frequency. Miss Dollbanell was immediately carried to bed and allowed to remain for a short time. In a quarter of an hour she was awakened, as on former days, by the mere will of her mesmeriser, in three or four seconds and at a distance of two meters.

She opened her eyes suddenly, smiled to those around her, and thus remained for about ten minutes without perceiving what had taken place, and free from all suffering. Then she said, without too strong an emotion, "Ah, I perceive it is over. What a blessing. Thanks, gentlemen."

Being requested to mention what she had felt or experienced during her sleep, she replied, "I know of nothing. I felt no pain. I recollect nothing." She was then asked how she knew that the operation had been performed.

Indicating the cradle used to elevate the bedclothes from the bed, she said, "Without that elevation above my knee, I should not have perceived it so soon, for I have no pain at this moment."

She was very calm the rest of the day and slept quietly the greater part of the night. It was the same the following days. On Monday, October 6th, the first bandages were removed at two o'clock and the wound dressed during mesmeric sleep. This dressing, which is generally very painful, gave her no sensation. On being awakened she had no knowledge of what had been done. From the moment of the operation (ten days had now elapsed) she constantly preserved a remarkable serenity and cheerfulness. She had not one bad symptom, not even the nervous excitement so common after painful operations. The wound is now nearly gradually healed, and there is every reason to hope for a speedy cure.

Today, October 13th, she left her room and took a turn in a neighboring garden and sat there afterwards for about two hours. She is now perfectly well and goes out every day.

The fourteenth day after the operation the wound was completely healed and all dressing left off. This amputation, performed under such extraordinary circumstances, and the rapid cure which ensued, have produced a strong sensation here.

O send out thy light and thy truth; let them lead me; let them bring me unto the holy hill, and to thy tabernacles.

(Psalms 43:3)

4 Life Energy Explorers

The written history of the human race points repeatedly to a basic and unshakable belief in some "quickening" or "enlivening" *influence* existing in the cosmos. This "subtle substance" has been referred to in various ways. It was called *vis animalis,* the Great Spirit, *vis naturalis,* and Prana. The French philosopher Henri Bergson postulated an *élan vital,* the electrical genius Nikola Tesla categorized it as "cosmic consciousness." The literature of mysticism is replete with references to this subtle, tenuous fluid that can penetrate walls, flesh, and all matter.

"Man," wrote Dr. Mesmer nearly two hundred years ago, "is immersed in an ocean of fluid, and it would be just as ridiculous to deny its existence as it would be for fish to deny that they exist in an ocean of water." It was this basic postulation of a Universal Fluid that underlay all of Mesmer's theoretical assumptions and formed the basis for his use of Animal Magnetism.

Until the objective, scientific verification of the existence of a pre-atomic, primordial, mass-free energy in the twentieth century by Wilhelm Reich, scientists lacked a firm scientific and clinical foundation for their postulates. Reich's discovery of the orgone is the most significant scientific breakthrough in man's history. The verified existence of a cosmic and biological energy will eventually demonstrate, as Reich often stated, that everyone is right in some way. We recall the poem about the blind men and the elephant: each man grabbed hold of a different part of the elephant—one touched the tusk; another, the tail; another felt the elephant's side—and then each concluded that the elephant was such-and-so, in accordance with his limited sensory knowledge.

One of the pioneering scientists who "grabbed hold" of the existence of a "magnetic fluid" was Baron Charles von Reichenbach, who is perhaps best known for his work as a chemist, and who gave the world creosote. Reichenbach was thoroughly familiar with Mesmer's work and therefore set out to establish the existence of Mesmer's "Universal Fluid." Although he published a considerable amount of material, his works are today very rare and difficult to obtain. He was reviewed often in Elliotson's *The Zoist,* and his most definitive work, covering a period from 1844 to 1847, published in London by Hippolyte Balliere in 1851, is titled: *Physico-Physiological Researches on the Dynamics of Magnetism, Electricity, Heat, Light, Crystallization and Chemism in their Relation to Vital Force.* This book, which I was privileged to read and review, was translated from the German by John Ashburner, M.D., another contributor to *The Zoist.*

Like Mesmer, Reichenbach can be considered a precursor of Wilhelm Reich; however, it is necessary to emphasize that the scientifically objective verification of the existence of a cosmic and biological energy belongs solely to Reich. The gathering of experimental data and the conducting of exhaustive tests—no matter how prolonged—do not in themselves constitute a bona fide scientific discovery. Until Reich, no one had been able to "isolate" the phenomenon, to verify it with thermometer, electroscope, Geiger counter, field meter, etc. And, what is equally important, no one was able to understand the basically different, *functional* laws of this hitherto "postulated" energy. The discovery of these basic laws, too, we owe to the arduous and dedicated labors of Wilhelm Reich.

Baron Reichenbach's researches, however, deserve consideration and should not be lost, and that is why I include a brief summation of the scope and thrust of his investigations. He became intrigued by Mesmer's published findings and thereafter set out to determine whether or not Mesmer's "pervasive force" could be objectified in his laboratory.

Beginning with the observation that certain "sensitives" were influenced by an iron magnet, he attempted to determine whether such persons could actually see any *light* coming from the poles of ordinary bar magnets or horseshoe magnets. Reichenbach saw a connection between the Aurora Borealis and mineral magnetism: since the aurora appeared like two streams of polarized light, perhaps the polarity of iron magnets might likewise "light up." His work with sensitive people brought the conclusion that there was indeed an "astonishing analogy" between the Aurora Borealis and the iron-magnetic emanations. He called this "force" the "Od."

Reichenbach's laboratory observations, made on a number of persons, indicated that magnets did indeed influence certain sensitive people. (This fact, we may recall, was never *denied* by Mesmer, who claimed, however, that the "force" did not originate in the magnets themselves but came from the atmosphere.) Reichenbach discovered that magnets "of 10-pounds supporting power," produced a rather unpleasant sensation on some persons when drawn along the body downwards without contact. Sensations were described as "like a warm wind," or "cooling, prickling, or creeping." In extremely sensitive patients, fainting, catalepsy, or violent spasms were induced.

One of Reichenbach's patients, described as a "cataleptic and spasmodic girl of twenty-five," and "whose vision made a dark room twilight to her," saw a "luminous appearance about the magnet." When the armature was removed from the magnet she "in profound darkness, saw a luminous appearance which uniformly disappeared when the armature was applied."

This woman was able to see, at a distance of ten feet, "a luminous vapor, surrounded by rays one-half to three-quarters of an inch long, constantly shooting and lengthening and shortening in the most beautiful manner from the poles." The light phenomenon always disappeared when the armature was applied, reappearing when it was removed. She described the light further as "almost purely white, sometimes mixed with iridescent colors, and denser towards the middle than towards the edges of the magnet."

The description of this "magnetic light" was repeated by many persons whom the Baron worked with, convincing him of the reality of this phenomenon. Reichenbach later described the various effects produced by crystals upon his patients. Crystals, like magnets, gave evidence of polarization. His patients distinguished two opposite points of the principal axes in these crystals: the minus or "north" pole, less powerful and "cool"; the plus or "south" pole, lukewarm. All agreed that they could distinguish *secondary* polar axes in these crystals. Reichenbach also noted that the "power" of a crystal could be transferred to solid bodies and water *by stroking them with one of its poles*. When crystals were only one and a half inches long, their power was scarcely perceptible. The power of the crystals increased in relation to their increased size.

Magnetic Meridian and Polarity

In the course of his work with patients, Reichenbach found that some persons were affected by their sleeping position in respect to terrestrial magnetism. For example, one individual usually awoke during the night and placed his head where his feet had been previously. If he did not change his sleeping position, this particular man found that "he was weary all day." Reichenbach found that when the man first went to bed, he lay with his head to the south and his feet to the north; after waking and changing positions, he lay with his head to the north and his feet to the south. Thereafter the man was advised to go to bed with his head facing north, and he found that he never had to change positions again.

Other patients showed similar sensitivity to position in relation to terrestrial magnetism, particularly if iron magnets were placed near them at the time. Reichenbach concluded that the general position of many of the sick during the use of magnets and mesmerism deserved serious consideration.

He further found that "magnetism" could be "collected" in a body. Again, in sensitive patients and those undergoing mesmerism, Reichenbach discovered that if he held a glass of water between his hands, such patients could distinguish the "magnetized water" from nonmagnetized water by smell, taste, et cetera. "All may object to this statement who have never investigated the matter," writes Reichenbach. "But all those who have investigated this subject can only speak with amazement. This water has received from the fingers and hand abundant charge of the peculiar force residing in them and retains this charge for some time."

Referring to the porality of the human body, Reichenbach found that placing the right hand in another person's left, or vice versa, produced considerably different results:

> When he placed his right hand in the patient's left, and his left hand simultaneously in her right, she described the sensation as of a perpetual current running up her right arm, across her breast and shoulders, down her left arm, and through him continually. It was painful and nearly caused her to faint. If now he crossed his hands, she could not endure it, and declared that there then arose so painful a sensation of a strange kind of struggle in her arms and through her breast (an undulation up and down the arm again) that she found it absolutely unendurable. After she released her hands she could not be persuaded to repeat the experiment.

Reichenbach concludes that in nervous cases it is "anything but indifferent which hand is given or taken—both hands are not in the same condition." This difference, the Baron concludes, can only be due to polarization. He believed that the main axis of man is *transverse*, that "we are formed of two symmetrical halves—everything, brain, organs, arms, hands, and feet are opposed to each other transversely, and it is especially transversely that we are polarized."

Reichenbach published the opinion that "Animal Magnetism has the following properties: it is conductable through other bodies; it may be communicated to other bodies either by directly charging them or by its dispersion. It soon disappears, but not immediately, from bodies charged with it. It assumes a polar arrangement in the animal body by virtue of its apparent dualism. It has no marked relation to the earth's magnetism. It attracts mechanically the hands of cataleptic patients, and its presence is associated with luminous phenomena."

Visual Evidence

Throughout the research of Mesmer and others who followed him, we come across descriptions of the "magnetic fluid" as observed by those undergoing mesmerism. Decimus Hands reported that one of his patients described the mesmeric fluid as "issuing from the ends of the fingers as clear streams of light, and quivering, resembling in color and brilliancy the rays of the sun." When passes were made upon this patient, she noted that this mesmeric fluid produced "a track, as of a phosphoric match that is struck in the dark." As the passes are continued, the mesmeric fluid appears to "load and illuminate the head and brain—these retain a dazzling, transparent brilliancy; the limbs are equally lit up, but they soon lose the brightness."

Mr. Hands questioned his patient critically when she spoke first about this "bright flame" that she saw issuing from the magnetizer's fingers and body. She said: "It is like smoke, like steam, like vapor—but no, it is distinctly different from each. I don't know what it is like. It resembles the phenomena often observable in a hayfield, from the currents of cold and hot air mingling—but the one mounting up, whilst the other is falling down. Or you may liken it to the mixing of spirits and water."

With respect to mesmerized water, this same patient described the fiery fluid as dropping "in quivering streams from the tips of my fingers to the bottom of the glass, til all the liquid was wholly illuminated, brilliant, and transparent."

Before all this is dismissed as the ravings of demented minds, it would be wise for the reader to examine a recent volume, *Psychic Discoveries Behind the Iron Curtain*, published in 1970.* Here the current work being done by distinguished Russian scientists, including actual photographs of the biological energy, fits precisely the descriptions given by mesmerized patients two centuries ago!

---

*By Sheila Ostrander and Lynn Schroeder (Englewood Cliffs, New Jersey. Prentice-Hall.)

Remarks by Dr. John Ashburner

Dr. John Ashburner, an eminent and skilled physician in his own right and translator of Reichenbach's voluminous experiments, was a regular contributor to Elliotson's *Zoist*, although he resided in the United States. The following remarks by Dr. Ashburner are germane to our discussion of the visualization of the magnetic fluid:

My patient described *a rope of blue light* proceeding from my eyes to her head whenever I willed her. She said it pulled so hard she could not resist it. She was obliged to approach me.

I have repeatedly asked her about the size of this "rope of light," and her answer was always that it was "in strings, in lines together, as thick as her arm, most frequently *blue*,* but sometimes all colors of the rainbow."

The magnetic sleep is induced by pointing two of my fingers to the eyes of this young woman. I have often produced the same kind of sleep by passing my hands alternately, at the distance of half-an-inch from the surface of her face and head, down from the crown of the head to the pit of the stomach, by darting my fingers at her face, by darting them at the nape of her neck, by standing before her and willing her to go to sleep—often even when she was unconscious of my doing it, as I showed before an audience at the Polytechnic Institute.

I have a right to infer that these effects are *produced by the emanation of a fluid from my person,* which has been seen by this person herself when I have mesmerized water. The *blue* streaks of light and the *blue* sparks from my fingers have been seen not by this patient alone but by other persons in a state of magnetic sleep *and by other persons, as*

---

*Blue and bluish-gray are specific colors of orgone energy.

well as by myself, in the ordinary condition of waking or
vigilance. That the exercise of thought is accompanied by
some emanation from the brain is manifest in this patient's
repeated observation of *"a blue cloud of light"* over my head
whenever I concentrated my mind in reading.

When another patient had lucidity enough to see me and
to know me for myself, she could see me dart *blue* sparks
into a glass of water whenever I mesmerized it. And if I
passed my hand over any other person, *that individual became quite clear to her.* [Apparently patients in the mesmeric
sleep are not able to make contact with anyone other than
the mesmerizer, unless such others are likewise "illuminated"
by magnetic passes. JE] If I willed, she saw blue streams of
light issue from my eyes. If I made passes rapidly down her
person, or down that of any other individual, she said she
saw a blue light, "in streaks" which resembled a beautiful
striped satin ribbon. Several of my patients in lucid mesmeric
sleep-waking have compared the appearance presented on
my making rapid passes to the very brilliantly colored blue
of satin striped ribbons.

A Final Word from Dr. Mesmer: Excerpts from
Memoir of 1799

It is only fitting, in concluding our review of the theory
and practice of Animal Magnetism, that we hear some final
remarks from the discoverer himself, Dr. Franz Anton Mesmer.

I had the honor in 1957 to bring out the first English
translation of Mesmer's *Memoir of 1799,* which gives the
basic, theoretical formulations that formed the foundation
of Mesmer's practice of Animal Magnetism. This volume,
published privately in limited edition, is long out of print.
Nevertheless, Dr. Mesmer's astute remarks and persuasive

observations still retain fresh thoughts for modern man. Let us now respectfully attend to some of Dr. Mesmer's remarks, derived from nearly a half century of observation, practice, and concentrated thought dealing with a subject to which he gave the fullest measure of his life as physician and humanitarian.

FROM *MEMOIR OF 1799*

History offers few examples of a discovery which, despite its importance, has experienced more difficulty in establishing itself than that of an agent acting upon the nervous system, an agent hitherto unknown which I call Animal Magnetism.

Philosophy is a newcomer in this age, triumphing over prejudice and superstition. It is particularly through ridicule that philosophy has succeeded in extinguishing the blazing fires of fanaticism and naiveté, because ridicule is an effective weapon against pride, and not easily resisted. Undoubtedly ridicule is the best means of changing opinion, if it is not used as an end in itself; but by an exaggerated zeal for philosophic progress, men very frequently abuse this means, and the most useful truths have thus been belittled, confused with the false, and rejected with them.

I set myself the task of investigating those ancient errors which have concealed the useful and the true. The ridiculousness and foolishness which cloak them must be separated from the original truths.

My first objective was to consider what might replace the absurd opinions that the destinies of men, as well as the events of nature, were supposed to be subject to the influence of the constellations and to different positions that heavenly bodies held to one another. The results of my meditations and research have produced a vast system of "influences" or of "communications" which connect all beings.

I am pleased to say that my discoveries will extend the boundaries of our knowledge of physics just as far as the invention of the microscope and telescope have done with respect to prior times. My discoveries will show that the health of man, as well as his existence, is based upon the general laws of nature; that man is endowed with a sensibility that places him in harmony with nature; that he possesses properties analogous to those of the magnet.

The phenomena which I have found in nature have led me to the common source of all things, and I believe my discoveries open a simple and correct route to truth and will redeem a large part of the study of the nature of metaphysical illusions.

There exists a universally diffused fluid, so continuous as not to allow of a vacuum, whose subtlety does not permit any comparison, and which by its very nature is able to receive, propagate, and communicate all impressions of movement.

One must compare the stubbornness of those who reject the idea of a *universal fluid* and the possibility of motion in solid matter to that of fish which would protest against one among them who proclaimed that the space between the bottom and the surface of the sea is filled by a fluid; that they live in this fluid; that it is only in this medium that they approximate and differ, one from the other, that enables them to contact one another, that connects them, and that this fluid is the sole means of their reciprocal relations!

It is therefore not permissible to doubt the existence of a universal fluid, which is nothing more than the basic mass of the entire range of matter. . . .

This fluid receives impressions and changes of movement, which it transmits, transfers, and applies to organized matter. My theory of influences will show how this universal fluid, without being heavy, causes what we call "gravity"; without being elastic, it cooperates in elasticity; in filling all space it brings about cohesion, without being in that condition itself.

As with all truths, it is impossible to progress in the study of nature without first having adopted her sequence of principles.

It is the *muscular fiber* which, by its particular mechanism, becomes the instrument of all movement. The streams of universal fluid are able to be applied to the intimate structures of muscular fiber exactly as wind or water acts upon a mill. The function of the muscular fiber—as moved by the universal fluid—consists in alternations of contraction and expansion, or relaxation. Contraction is a positive action, and this faculty of contraction and expansion is called *irritability*.

The action of expansion and contraction upon the vessels containing liquid is the cause of the circulation of the body. The defect of either contraction or expansion checks the stream. As soon as the bodily fluids are deprived of local and internal movement, they thicken and consolidate. Such thickening or cessation of the fluids extends to a more or less considerable extent.

Another result of the cessation of the movement of the fluids is their *degeneration*. When the flow of fluids is stopped or slackened in the vessels, this condition is called *obstruction*.

The muscular fiber, animated by the principle of irritability, is again susceptible to an internal influence, which is called *irritation*. The effect of this influence is the contraction of the fiber.

Every action of the muscular fiber may be considered as dependent wholly upon either irritability or irritation. Consequently, there are two causes of obstructions: first, when a vessel had lost its ability to contract (irritability); second, when a vessel is in a state of irritation, or when it meets with some obstacle to its dilation. Therefore, in both cases, the conditions necessary for the alternating action of vessels have been thwarted and their action stopped.

Without going into the details of this aberration, which is almost general and all but restricted to living matter, it is easy to conceive, according to a general law, that an impulse toward movement is always met by a resisting effort, and that the impulse toward movement must be adjusted so that it overcomes the resisting effort. This effort is called *crisis*, and all the effects which result directly from this crisis are called *critical symptoms*. They are the true means of recovery, or what constitutes *the natural cure;* whereas the effects stemming from the resistance to this natural effort are called *symptomatic symptoms*. These produce what is called the *illness*.

The crisis is determined by the irritation of the fiber from which it is provoked, be it through the intension of irritability, by an increased effort on the resisting fiber, or finally by the meeting of these two causes.

None of the aberrations within the animal body can be remedied without having experienced the effects of the effort —that is to say, each illness cannot be cured without a crisis.

Hippocrates seems to have been the first and perhaps the only one who grasped the phenomena of crises in critical diseases. He recognized that the different symptoms were only modifications of the efforts which nature makes against diseases. After him, however, whenever men observed the same symptoms in chronic illnesses, far removed from their initial causes, and without the fever attendant upon critical diseases, they isolated these symptoms, fabricated many "diseases," and characterized each *with a different name*.

Instead of being distracted by the most diverse symptoms, Hippocrates predicted the cure. His assurance was based upon his daily observation of the progress of the disease, which he called *critiques*. He vaguely sensed the existence of an external and general element by which the action of the disease was being regulated.

What the father of medicine had observed, and what others after him have called nature, are only the effects of the element which I have discovered and whose existence I have announced: an element which can solve for us the nature of ebb and flow, or the intension and remission of matter.

It is regrettable that the light Hippocrates flashed upon the healing art was restricted to acute illnesses. He might have realized that chronic diseases differ from others only by the continuity and rapidity with which the symptoms succeed each other. Acute illnesses are to chronic illnesses as the life of an ephemeral insect is to the life of other animals. Insects undergo in twenty-four hours all the changes of age, sex, growth and decline, while other animals take years to pass through the same conditions.

Furthermore, it is regrettable that medicine still ignores, for the most part, the natural and necessary development of chronic diseases: it opposes them by the use of drugs which disturb their progress, arrest their course, and frequently bring on premature death.

The progress and development of epilepsy, for example, as well as manic and melancholy cases, of swollen glands and their complications, of affected sense organs—all are still generally unknown, and it is chiefly in these illnesses that we confuse the crisis with the disease.

The immediate cause of all disease, internal or external, implies the defect or irregularity of the circulation of the humors, or *obstructions* of different kinds of vessels. As I have stated, we shall finally understand that such conditions arise as the result of a default of *irritability*, or of the action of solids upon the humors they contain; that instead of having to resort to innumerable assortments of specifics and drugs, we have only two functions to perform: (1) *to know how to reestablish the irritability or action of solids upon liquids; (2) to know how to forestall and prevent any impediment which opposes such irritability or action.*

It has been proven and established through the system of influences, and through exact observation, that the large celestial bodies partially control the movement of our planet. The ebb and flow common to the earth's component parts, life, the process of fermentation, and the general and particular rotations to which the earth is susceptible, are all naturally determined by that influence, which, by the means of *the continuity of a universal fluid,* produces an increase or reduction of all material properties, as one can see in the growth and decline of vegetation.

It is thus by the same causes that irritability (in the muscular fiber) is naturally increased or diminished, so that the development of diseases and their cure are regulated and determined by that influence, or by what I call *natural magnetism.*

How this natural effect, though general, can only become useful to certain persons who are particularly disposed to it remains for me to discover. I believe, however, that I have discovered in nature that the mechanism of influences consists of a type of reciprocal and alternating *flow* of "streams" coming and going, and that these streams consist of the subtle substance that fills all space. It is impossible to cause a displacement of this subtle substance without a corresponding replacement taking place. Thus, if a movement of the subtle substance is provoked within a body, there immediately occurs a similar movement in another sensitive to receiving it, whatever the distance between the two persons.

Animal Magnetism, considered as an agent, is thus an effective "invisible fire"—it is a question of:

1. Knowing how to provoke and maintain this fire by every possible means, and of applying it.

2. Understanding and clearing away the obstacles which disturb or impede its action and the gradual effect which one tries to obtain in treatment.

3. Understanding and anticipating the course of development in order to steadfastly adjust oneself to maintaining treatment until cure is established.

Thus, in a general and concise form, we have the discovery of Animal Magnetism, which can be regarded as a *means* of preventing and curing disease.

Considering that the reciprocal influence is general between all bodies; that the *magnet* represents the model of that universal law, and that the animal body is susceptible to properties analogous to the magnet, I feel sufficiently justified in using the name *animal magnetism*, which I have adopted to designate the system or doctrine of influences in general, giving it suitability to the animal body as well as to the remedy and method of cure.

Life in all creatures in the universe is one and the same: it consists of the movement of the most subtle substance. Death is repose, or the cessation of motion. The natural and inevitable course of life consists in passing through the state of fluidity to that of solidity.

Man is endowed with the faculty of perception. By means of sensations and their effects, he is in rapport with other substances and living beings outside himself. The various sense organs render him capable of experiencing the effects of the different material which surround him. The principle which animates and causes him to act is determined by sensations; and all actions are the result of sensations.

Apart from the known organs, we also have other organs

able to receive sensations. We cannot doubt their existence because of their ability to take in the most delicate impressions; and there are strong reasons to believe that we are endowed with an *internal* sense which is related to the whole universe, and which can be considered as an *extension* of sight.

According to my theory of crises, and in observing the neglected development of chronic diseases, I have identified the phenomenon I call "critical sleep," whose changes were easily and frequently observed by me and opened a new field to my observations on the nature of man.

Man's sleep is not a negative state, nor is it simply the absence of wakefulness: modifications of that state have proven that the faculties of a sleeping man continue to function, often with more perfection than when he is awake.

In that sleeping state of crisis, there are persons who are able to foresee the future and bring the most remote things into present time. *Their senses can extend to every distance and in all directions,* without being checked by obstacles. In brief, it appears that all nature is known to them. *Even the will may be communicated to them,* apart from conventional means. These faculties differ in each individual. The more common phenomenon consists of *being able to see the interior of their bodies, as well as those of others, and of judging accurately the nature of diseases, their progress, the necessary treatment, and the results.** But it is rare to find all these faculties combined in any one individual.

The perfection of this critical sleep varies according to the progress and duration of crisis, as well as by the character, temperament, and habits of the patients—but particularly by a kind of education that we give them in this state, and

---

*This ability was demonstrated in thousands of "readings" given by Edgar Cayce.

by the manner in which we direct their faculties. In this regard we can compare our patients to a telescope, in which the effects vary according to the way we adjust it.

It is essential to mention that all kinds of mental derangements are only gradations of an imperfect sleep. It is therefore of extreme importance to distinguish between *the symptomatic* and *the critical sleep* of diseases.

From my principles and developments, it follows that ancient beliefs cannot be disregarded simply because they are associated with error. The phenomenon of somnambulism has been known in every age and perverted according to the principles of each. The extraordinary faculties of the somnambulistic patient have never been properly regarded as *the extension of his sensations and instinct.*

More important than the obstacles which have been thrown in my way, I have believed it necessary to progress to publish my ideas. I voluntarily surrender my theory to criticism, declaring that I have neither the time nor the desire to reply to it. I have nothing to say to those who are incapable of crediting me with integrity or generosity, and who cannot substitute anything better for that of mine which they seek to destroy.

I would regard with pleasure any better inspirations which might bring forth sounder, more enlightened principles—some talent better understood than mine, which might discover new facts and perhaps make my doctrine even more beneficial by new conceptions and work. In brief, I wish that someone might go further than I have gone.*

As for my fame, it will always be sufficient that I have been able to open a vast new field for the considerations of

---

*This hope was to be fulfilled in the twentieth-century by the discoveries of Dr. Wilhelm Reich.

science, and have, to some extent, outlined the route of this new course.

Although I am rather advanced in years, I wish to dedicate my remaining life to the sole practice of a method that I have discovered to be eminently useful in the preservation of my fellowman, in order that hereafter they might not be further exposed to the incalculable hazards of the application of drugs.

FRANZ ANTON MESMER, Doctor of Medicine

5 *Maxims on Animal Magnetism*

Chapter 1: Principles

1. God exists as an uncreated source. In Nature two created sources exist: matter and movement.

2. Primary matter is that which has been employed by the Creator for the formation of all beings.

3. Movement brings about the development of all possibilities.

4. We have not yet formed a positive idea of the primary matter; it is placed between the simple being [or simplest thing formed, Ed.] and the beginning of the composed being. It is like unity with regard to arithmetic quantities.

5. Impenetrability constitutes the essence of primary matter; impenetrability belongs to it alone, and to none other.

6. Matter is indifferent to being in movement or in repose.

7. Matter in movement constitutes fluidity; the cessation of movement in matter produces solidity.

8. If two or more parts of matter are in repose, a combination results from this state.

9. The condition of the combination is a condition relative to the movement or repose of matter.

10. Only in these relations is found the source of all possible variations, in forms and in properties.

11. Since matter is capable only of different combinations, ideas that we have concerning numbers or arithmetic quantities can serve to make us aware of the immensity of developmental possibilities.

12. Considering the particles of the elementary matter as units, one can easily realize that these units can assemble themselves by two's, by three's, by four's, five's, etc., and that such assemblages will result in sums or aggregates which can be continued to infinity.

13. The manner of assemblage of these units into aggregates constitutes the first species of possible combinations.

14. Considering then these first combinations as new units, we will have as many species of units as there will be numbers possible, and we will be able to conceive also of assemblages of these units among themselves.

15. If these assemblages or aggregates are formed of units of the same species, they constitute the whole of *homogeneous matter*.

16. If these aggregates are formed of units of different species, they constitute the whole of *heterogeneous matter*.

17. From these diverse combinations, by which each can proceed to infinity, one can conceive of the immensity of all possible combinations.

18. Properly speaking, the elementary matter does not have, by itself, any property. It is indifferent to being in any type of combination; and all properties which it presents to us are the result or product of its diverse combinations.

19. The whole of a quantity of matter, which becomes and is regarded as forming a combined entity, is that which we call a *body*.

20. If in the combination of the constituent parts of a body, there exists an order, in consequence of which there results

new effects, or new combinations, such a unit is called an *organic body*.

21. If the parts of matter are combined in such an order, from which there results no new effect, or new combination, the resultant unit is called an *inorganic body*.

22. What we call an *inorganic body* is purely a metaphysical distinction because if there were absolutely no effect of a body, it would not exist.

23. The elementary matter of all the constituent parts of bodies is of the same nature. This identity is proven in the final dissolution of bodies.

24. If we consider the constituent parts of bodies as existences, separate from one another, we have the idea of *locality*.

25. Locations are imaginary points in which matter is found or can be found.

26. The quantity of these imaginary points determines the idea of *space*.

27. If the matter changes location, and occupies successively different points, this change or this action of matter is what we call *movement*.

28. Movement modifies matter.

29. The first movement is an immediate effect of creation, and this movement supplied to the matter is the sole cause of all the different combinations and all the forms which exist.

30. This movement is constantly and universally maintained by the most tenuous parts of the matter which we call *fluid*.

31. We shall consider three things in all movements of the fluid matter: the *direction*, the *speed*, and the *tone*.

32. The tone is the kind or mode of movement which maintains its material parts in a specific condition.

33. There are only two directions, and these are directly opposed, one to the other. All other directions are composed of these two; by one of these directions the parts approach

each other, and by the other they diverge. Combination occurs through the one; the other results in dissolution.

34. Equality in the force of these two directions causes the
parts neither to approach nor to diverge from each other;
consequently, they are neither in the state of cohesion nor
dissolution, but are in the state which constitutes perfect
fluidity.

35. To the extent that the two directions diverge from the
state of equality, the fluidity diminishes and solidity increases, and *vice versa*.

36. Combination or primary cohesion takes place when the
directions of movement of the parts happen to oppose one
another, or when their speed toward the same direction is
unequal.

37. A quantity of matter in the state of cohesion or of rest
constitutes the solidity or the mass of bodies.

38. The first impulse to movement which the matter has received in an absolutely filled space is sufficient to give it all
the directions and all the gradations of speed possible.

39. Matter conserves the quantity of movement that it has
received initially.

40. The different kinds of movement can be considered either
in the entire body or in the constituent parts.

41. The constituent parts of the fluid matter can be combined in all possible ways, and can receive all kinds of movement possible among themselves.

42. All the properties may be organized or unorganized, depending upon the manner in which their parts are combined,
and the movement of these parts among themselves.

43. If a quantity of fluid is set in motion in one direction, that
is called a *current*.

44. If we suppose a current which insinuates itself into a
body, dividing itself into an infinite number of small currents,

infinitely tenuous, in a pattern of lines, we call these subdivisions *streams*.

45. When the elementary matter, either by moving in opposing directions, or at unequal speeds, sets itself at rest, and thereby acquires some cohesion, from the way in which the particles are combined there results some spaces or *interstices*.

46. The interstices or masses remain permeable to the currents or streams of the subtle matter.

47. All bodies submerged in a fluid are obedient to the movement of that fluid.

48. It follows that if a body is submerged in a current, it is drawn along in its direction, which does not happen to a body obeying several mixed directions.

49. Given A——C——B——:

If A moves toward B, and if the cause of movement is B, this would make for what we call attraction. If A moves in B, and if the cause of movement is C, then this would make for what we call mechanical driving, or *apparent attraction*.

50. The cause of the apparent attraction and repulsion is in the direction of currents coming and going.

51. When the streams of opposing currents impose upon one another immediately, there is attraction; when they collide with each other in opposition, there is repulsion.

52. Considering that all is one whole, there cannot exist an incoming current without an outgoing current, and *vice versa*.

53. Within the universe there exists a fixed, uniform, and constant amount of movement, which was impressed upon matter in the beginning.

54. This impression of movement was made upon one mass of fluid at first, so that all the contiguous parts of fluid have received the same impressions.

55. It resulted in two opposed directions, and in all the progressions of other composed movements.

56. Given (A) (B), all being one whole, if A moves towards B, it may mean two things: that B was displaced by A, and A was replaced by B.

57. This figure explains: (1) all the gradations and directions of movement; (2) a movement of universal and particular rotation; (3) that this movement is only propagated for a certain distance from the first impression; (4) that currents, both universal and particular, are more or less composed; and

58. (5) by means of these currents, the sum of movement is distributed and applied to all parts of matter.

59. There exists within the modification of the currents the source of all the combinations and of all the movements possible, developed and to be developed. Thus, in the infinite number of combinations of matter, as the movement of one or another type may have brought about by chance, those combinations which might be considered perfect (that is to say, where there is no degree of contradiction of movement), have subsisted and are conserved, and in perfecting themselves have succeeded in forming the matrices for the propagation of the species. One can gain an idea of this operation by comparing it with crystallizations.

60. All bodies are floating in a current of the subtle matter [that is, the universal fluid (Ed.)].

61. Thus it is that by the opposition of directions, and unequal speeds, the particles touch each other. They are left thereby without movement, and form the first degree of cohesion. An infinity of molecules more gross are induced and applied more extensively to the first [cohesed particle (Ed.)], all of which are at rest and constitute a mass which becomes the germ and origin of all large bodies.

62. Two particles which are at rest constitute an obstacle to

the two streams of currents which correspond to them. Being unable to pass with integrity, these two streams join together with two adjacent streams and accelerate their movement, and this acceleration is due to the passages' or interstices' [of the particles (Ed.)] being more restricted.

63. Upon approaching a solid body, every current is accelerated, and this acceleration occurs by virtue of the compactibility of the matter.

64. These streams either retain or lose their initial direction in passing, and thus their parts may follow a confused movement.

65. If this current, in traversing a body, is split into two separate streams, and if the opposing fibers [of the body (Ed.)] split in two, the streams insinuate themselves mutually into the interstices of each, without disturbing their motion; the result is apparent attraction, or the phenomenon of the magnet.

66. If instead of insinuating themselves, the streams collide so that one predominates over the other, the result is repulsion.

67. Equilibrium demands that when a current enters into a body, another equal to it flows out of it, and yet the movement of the departing streams may be weaker, because they are divergent and scattered.

68. The nature of the universal and particular streams being thus determined, one can account for the origin and progress of celestial bodies.

69. (1) The coarsest molecule which chance has formed, let us say, has become the center of a particular current.

70. (2) The current, in proportion to its involvement of the floating molecule which it surrounds, has enlarged this central body. Thus the current becomes accelerated and more all-encompassing, taking to itself coarser matter. This action is extended to a distance where the current finds itself coun-

ter-balanced by the similar action from another central body.

71. (3) As the action is produced equally from the periphery to the center, the bodies necessarily become *spheres*.

72. (4) The difference of their mass depends upon the random combination of the first molecules, which gives them greater or lesser size.

73. (5) The differences of their mass corresponds to the extent of the space which is found between them.

74. (6) As all matter has received a movement of rotation, there results in each central body a movement upon its axis.

75. (7) As these bodies are relatively eccentric to the whirl-pool in which they are submerged, they move away from the center up to the point where the centrifugal movement is proportionate to the force of the current which carries them towards the center.

76. (8) All celestial bodies have a reciprocal tendency towards each other, in proportion to their mass and distance: this action is most directly exercised between the points of their surfaces which face each other.

77. (9) These spherical bodies turning upon their axes, and reciprocally exposing to each other one-half of their surfaces, receive mutual impressions upon that half. These mutual and alternative impressions constitute the ebb and flow in each of their spheres.

78. (10) These actions and these reciprocally described relationships constitute the influence between all celestial bodies. They are manifested in more remote bodies by the effects which they produce upon each other. They disturb one another in their revolutions; they arrest, retard, or accelerate the movement of each other's orbits.

79. (11) Hence there is a constant law in nature, that there is a mutual influence upon the totality of bodies, and consequently this influence exerts itself upon all the constituent parts and their properties.

80. This reciprocal influence and the relations of all co-existent bodies form what is called *magnetism*.

Chapter 2: On Cohesion

81. Cohesion is the state of matter in which its particles exist together in local movement and are not able to free themselves without an external effort.

82. The matter can attain cohesion through directly opposed movement, or by the inequality of speed in the same direction.

83. Two particles which touch each other exclude the subtle matter [universal fluid (Ed.)] at the point of contact; separation cannot be made without an effort against the subtle matter which surrounds them, and the effort necessary to bring this about must be equal to the resistance.

84. The resistance is equal to the entire column which comes up to the point of contact.

85. The total resistance occurs only momentarily, at the instant of separation.

86. Resistance or cohesion is therefore to be considered as combining the points of contact and the weight of the column of universal fluid in which the body is submerged: the column being based upon the points of contact.

87. The column upon the resisting matter is invariable, and cohesion occurs by virtue of the points of contact.

88. Since cohesion exists only at such times as the continuity of the fluid is interrupted by contact, as soon as the continuity is reestablished, cohesion ceases.

Chapter 3: On Elasticity

89. A body is elastic when, after compression, it reestablishes itself in its former state.

90. Elasticity in bodies is the property of reestablishing them-

selves in their former state after having been compressed.
91. A body is therefore elastic:

1—When the parts which compose it can, by their shape, be brought together or drawn apart, without being displaced among themselves;

2—When these same particles can withstand an effort to discontinue their cohesion, without such effort being sufficient to bring it about;

In the first case—that is, when the molecules are compressed, the streams of the subtle fluid are narrowed without being discontinued, and thus act as so many wedges upon the lateral surfaces of the molecules, with all the more force, since their speed has been increased by the narrowing of the interstices.

In the second case, an effort is made to overcome the moment of cohesion; this effort, being insufficient, continues until it is overcome and exhausted by the cohesion.

92. The compressed elastic body, at the instant of compression, is able to bear the resistance to cohesion without being entirely overcome. It is the moment of resistance to the greatest effort that just falls short of initiating a separation which constitutes the highest degree of elasticity of a body. In this state, it withstands the action of the column of fluid —that is to say that the effort brought about to overcome cohesion is equal to the action of the column of fluid pressing upon the lateral surfaces of the molecules, and [the effort] must lift that column in order to overcome its action.

93. The more an elastic body is compressed, the more the resistance is increased; the cause of elasticity being, in part, due to cohesion, the resistance is a factor of the quantity of the points of contact upon which the efforts are being brought to bear, and which are opposing these efforts.

94. Nonelastic bodies are those in which the compressed

parts can, by their shapes, be displaced without being discontinued among themselves.

95. In an elastic body the parts cannot displace each other without the dissolution of cohesion.

96. The gradations of efforts against cohesion and the gradations of resistance to the cause of cohesion produce all the effects of elasticity.

97. These efforts give to the constituent parts another direction, without being able to dissolve them. The constituent parts move in relation to each other, without leaving their place [in the whole (Ed.)].

Chapter 4: On Gravity

98. There is a reciprocal tendency among all coexistent bodies. This tendency is in consideration of masses and distances.

99. The causes of this reciprocal tendency are the currents in which these bodies are found to be submerged, and in which the strength and quantity of movement depends upon the composite factors of their mass, their size, and their speed.

100. It is this tendency that we call gravity, whereby all the coexistent bodies gravitate toward each other.

101. A general current of the subtle elementary matter [fluid (Ed.)] is directed toward the center of our globe and draws along in its direction all of the combined matter which it encounters, and which by their composition present a resistance to the fluid.

102. In principle, there results towards a center a precipitation of all the particles which are found within the entire extent of the activity of this current, in the order of their resistance, so that any material which is more gross would present the greater resistance and would precipitate first.

103. In this way all the layers of matter, which compose different globes, are formed.

104. The moving force being applied to each of the particles of the original combinations, the quantitative gravitational effect is in consideration of the speed of the current and the resistance of the matter.

105. As the speed of the currents increases in approaching the earth, gravity increases in the same proportion.

106. The earth gravitates equally towards all heavy bodies and towards all the constituent particles.

107. Within the points where the currents are found in equilibrium, gravity ceases.

108. At a certain depth of the earth's mass, gravity ceases.

109. Those fluids which are capable of changing the *compactibility* of combined matter, and those which are capable of changing the intensity of currents, can also increase or decrease the gravity of bodies. Such fluids are capable also of a change of movement, rotation, a variation in the cause of ebb and flow, calcination, and vitrification.

110. The causes and modifications of gravity are also the causes for the variations of material solidity of the earth's constituent parts.

111. The solidity or *compactibility* of the earth increases to a certain depth, after which it probably diminishes.

Chapter 5: On Fire

112. There are two directions of movement. By virtue of one, the parts of the matter approach each other, and by virtue of the other they depart from each other. The former is the principle of combination; the latter affects dissolution.

113. An extremely rapid, oscillatory movement of the matter, which is directed at a body whose combination [molecular (Ed.)] is found to be at a certain degree of cohesion, produces in that body a dissolution, which is fire.

114. Considered in relation to our senses, fire produces an oscillatory movement upon the universal fluid, which, being propagated to the retina, represents the idea of the *flame*, or glow of fire, and being reflected by other bodies represents the idea of light.

115. This same movement propagated and applied to the parts destined for the sense of touch, in diminishing or weakening cohesion more or less, presents the idea of *warmth*.

116. The state of fire is therefore a state of matter which is opposed to the state of cohesion and is therefore a condition which can, more or less, diminish the cohesion of matter.

117. Phlogistic matter is one which, by virtue of its delicate combination, cannot resist the action of the opposing movement.

118. Combustibility occurs by virtue of the delicate quality of matter. The different gradations of the movement and reconciliation toward the state of fire produce the various degrees of heat and their effects.

Chapter 6: On Ebb and Flow

119. The cause of the gravity of all large bodies is also the cause of all the properties of organized and unorganized bodies.

120. The rotating motion of the spheres and their different distances occur because of the mutual influence being applied successively and alternately to those parts of the globes which are in opposition to one another.

121. The surface of the globe is covered by liquid matter, *the atmosphere and water,* which conform to the laws of hydrostatics and equilibrium.

122. The part which assumes this general aspect, having lost its gravity, the lateral parts compress and raise this portion, until it establishes equilibrium with the rest. The surface of the atmosphere and of the sea therefore become a spheroid,

the longer axis of which is turned toward the moon, and follows in its course. In this operation the sun cooperates, although more feebly.

123. We call this alternative effect of gravitational principles, ebb and flow.

124. When different causes [of ebb and flow (Ed.)] converge, be it relative to diverse stars or to the earth in which this action becomes common to all the constituent parts and to all the beings which occupy them, might there not be an ebbing and flowing which is more or less individual or composed?

125. The effects of this alternative and reciprocal action, which increase and decrease the properties of organized and unorganized bodies, are called *intension and remission*. Thus by this action, cohesion, gravity, electricity, elasticity, Magnetism, and irritability are increased or decreased.

126. In regard to the respective opposition of the earth and the moon, this action is strongest during the equinoxes:

127. (1) Since the centrifugal tendency upon the equator is more considerable, the gravity of the waters and of the atmosphere is thus weaker.

128. (2) Since the action of the sun concurs with that of the moon, this action is again the stronger when the moon is in the sign of Boreas, when it is in opposition, or in conjunction, with the sun.

129. The diverse concourse of these causes modifies the intension of ebb and flow in different ways.

130. Just as all the particular bodies upon the surface of the earth have their mutual influence or tendency, there also exists a special cause of ebb and flow.

131. Independent of the ebb and flow just presented, there are cycles of ebb and flow according to ages, years, months, days, and various others, irregular and accidental.

Chapter 7: On Electricity

132. If two masses whose surfaces are charged by unequal quantities of movement meet each other, they communicate the surplus charge in order to achieve equilibrium. The lesser charged mass receives the surplus charge from the greater. This discharge is made either by a considerable quantity at an instant, or successively, in the manner of streams.

The first case manifests itself by an explosion capable of producing the phenomena of *fire* and of *sound*.

The second case produces the effects of apparent attraction and repulsion. The product of these effects is called *electricity*. The effects observed in nature are called natural electricity. It occurs in clouds through unequal heat, or even between the clouds and the earth.

133. The surplus of movement excited by the friction of an elastic body which happens to be exposed to another body so as to effect a discharge forms *artificial electricity*.

134. In all electrical phenomena we observe currents coming and going.

Chapter 8: On Man

135. By virtue of his constitution, man may be considered in a state of sleep, in a state of wakefulness, in a state of health, or in a state of sickness. In man, as in all of nature, there are only two principles: matter and movement.

136. The material mass of which man consists can be increased or decreased.

137. Since any decrease must be restored, the lost matter is therefore replenished to the general mass by means of food.

138. The lost quantity of movement is restored by the sum

of the general movement [in which man is immersed (Ed.)] through sleep.

139. Just as man has two kinds of energy losses, in like manner does he have two ways of restoration—through food and sleep.

140. In the state of sleep, man acts like a machine in which the sources of movement are internal.

141. The state of man's sleep is one in which the exercise and function of a considerable part of his being are suspended for a time, during which the quantity of movement lost while awake is restored by means of the properties of the universal currents in which he is immersed.

142. There are two kinds of universal currents relative to man: gravity, and the magnetic current from one pole to the other.

143. Man receives and collects a certain quantity of movement, as in a reservoir. The surplus or fullness of the reservoir induces wakefulness.

144. Man begins his existence in the state of sleep. In this state the amount of movement that he receives proportionate to his mass is employed in the formation and development of the rudiments of his organs.

145. As soon as that formation is achieved, he wakes up, producing rather powerful efforts upon his mother, in order to bring about his birth.

146. Man is in a state of health when all the parts of which he is composed are able to exercise the functions for which they are destined.

147. If perfect order rules all of his functions, one calls this state the state of *harmony*.

148. Sickness is the opposite state—that is to say, one wherein harmony is disturbed.

149. Just as there is only one harmony, there is only one health.

150. Health is represented by the straight line.

151. Illness is the aberration of this line, this aberration being more or less considerable.

152. The *remedy* is the means that reestablishes the order or harmony which has been disturbed.

153. The principle which constitutes, restores, and maintains harmony is the principle of conservation: the principle of cure is therefore necessarily the same.

154. The portion of the universal movement which man received as his original share, and which was initially modified in the womb, becomes tonic, and determines his formation and the development of the viscera and all the other constituent organic parts.

155. That portion of movement is the source of his life.

156. This source maintains and rectifies the function of all the viscera.

157. The viscera are the constituent organic parts which prepare, rectify, and assimilate all their humors—determining movement, secretions, and excretions.

158. The living source [of movement (Ed.)], being a part of the universal movement and obeying the laws common to the universal fluid, is therefore submissive to all the impressions of the influence of celestial bodies, of the earth, and of the particular bodies which surround it.

159. This faculty or property of man of being susceptible to all these relations is what we call *Magnetism*.

160. Man, being continuously surrounded by universal and individual currents, is affected by them; the movement of the universal fluid becomes modified by the varying structure of his constituent parts and becomes tonic. In this tonic state it follows the continuity of the body and moves toward the most prominent parts.

161. From these prominences or extremities, the tonic currents flow away and rejoin the atmospheric currents. This

occurs more readily when a body capable of receiving or conveying them is placed in opposition to such extremities. When this occurs, the currents become restricted into a point and their speed is increased.

162. The points of outlet or entrance of tonic currents are what we call *poles*. These poles are analogous to those which we observe in the magnet.

163. The poles can therefore destroy or increase the currents which are entering or departing, as in a magnet: their communication is the same. It is sufficient to determine only one pole, since the opposite pole is formed at the same time.

164. On an imaginary line between the two poles there is a center or point of equilibrium where the action is nullified —that is, where neither direction predominates.

165. These currents can be propagated and communicated to a considerable distance, be it through the continuity or series of bodies or through that of a fluid, like air and water.

166. All bodies whose shapes terminate at a point or angle serve to receive the currents and become *conductors*.

167. The apertures of foramens or of canals which serve as passageways can be regarded as conductors for the currents.

168. Always preserving the tonic character which they have received, these currents can penetrate all solid and liquid bodies.

169. These currents can be communicated and propagated by every means where continuity exists—be it solid, fluid, in the rays of light, or through the continuity of the oscillations of sound.

170. The currents can be reinforced:

171. (a) Through all the causes of ordinary movement—such as internal and local motions, sounds, noises, the wind, electric and all other friction, and through bodies which already are endowed with movement, like the magnet, or through living bodies

172. (b) Through their communication with heavy bodies, in which they can be collected and concentrated as in a reservoir, to be distributed later in different directions

173. (c) Through the quantity of bodies to which the currents are communicated—the elemental current* not having mass, but rather being a modification, its effect increases like that of fire, to the extent to which it is communicated.

174. If the current of the Magnetism concurs in its direction with the general current, or with the Magnetic current of the earth, the general result is an increase of intensity of all these currents.

175. These currents can also be reflected in mirrors, according to the laws of light.

Chapter 9: On Sensations

176. To perceive is a property of organized matter: the faculty of receiving impressions.

177. As the body forms itself through the continuity of matter, thus sensations result from the continuity of the impressions or affections of the organized body.

178. This continuity of affections constitutes a whole, a unity, which can combine, arrange, compare, modify, and organize itself; and the result of this is a thought.

179. Any change in the proportions and in the relation of affections of our body produces a thought which could not otherwise have been produced.

180. This thought represents the difference between the former state and the altered state—the sensation, therefore, being the perception of such alteration; and the sensation is in consideration of the difference.

---

*Mesmer is referring here to the universal fluid—the primary, mass-free "stuff" of life, scientifically verified as "orgone energy" by Dr. Wilhelm Reich.

181. There are as many sensations possible as there are possible differences among the proportions.

182. The instruments or organs which serve to perceive the differences of affections are called the *senses*. The principal constituent parts of these organs in all animals are the nerves, which, in greater or lesser quantity, are exposed to being affected by different orders of matter.

183. In addition to the known organs, we also have other organs proper to receiving impressions. We cannot doubt of their existence, but because of our habitual use of our known organs in such a predominant manner, and because of the strong impressions to which we have accustomed ourselves, we do not allow ourselves to perceive more delicate impressions.

184. It is very likely, and there are strong *a priori* reasons, that we are endowed with an internal sense which is in communication with the entire universe. With it we are able to understand the possibility of presentiments.

185. If it is possible to be affected in such a way as to have the idea of a being at an infinite distance—just as we are able to see stars by way of impressions conveyed to us in a straight line through the succession of a material substance coexistent with them and our organs of sight—why should it not be possible to be affected by objects whose successive movement is propagated to us in curved or oblique lines, and from any direction? Why should we not be affected by the chain of beings which succeed each other?

186. One law of sensation is that in all the affections which are brought to bear upon our organs, the stronger becomes sensible. The stronger sensation effaces the weaker.

187. We cannot sense an object as it really is but only the impression it makes, depending upon the nature and disposition of the organ which receives such impression, and the impressions which have preceded it.

188. Our sensations, therefore, are the result of all the affects to which our organs are subject.

189. Furthermore, we can understand that our senses cannot represent objects as they are; we can only approximate, more or less, the knowledge as to the nature of objects, through usage and application, combined and reflected by the different senses, but we can never reach their full truth.

Chapter 10: On Instinct

190. The faculty of feeling the connection within the universal harmony which creatures and events have to the conservation of each individual is what we should call *instinct*.

191. All animals are endowed with this faculty. It is subject to the common laws of sensations. This sensation is stronger in proportion to the concern which events manifest upon our preservation.

192. Sight is an example of a sense by which we can perceive the connections which coexistent beings have among themselves, as well as their relations and actions upon us, insofar as they affect us directly.

193. This relation or difference of interest is to instinct what height and distance are to sight.

194. Because this instinct is an effect of order, of harmony, it becomes a sure criterion of actions and sensations; it is solely a question of cultivating and maintaining this chief sensibility.

195. A man insensible to instinct is like an angle in regard to invisible objects.

196. The man who can only use what he calls reason is like one who uses glasses to examine everything which might come into his view; he becomes habitually disposed not to see with his own eyes and can never see objects as others see them.

197. Instinct is natural; reason is artificial. Every man arrives at his own reason, but instinct is a determined and invariable result of the order of nature upon each individual.

198. Man's life consists of that portion of the universal movement which, initially becoming tonic and applied to one bit of matter, has been directed to form organs and viscera and then to support and rectify their functions.

199. Death is the complete abolition of tonic movement. Man's life begins by movement and ends by repose. Just as in all nature movement is the source of combinations and of repose, likewise in man the principle of life becomes the cause of death.

200. All development and formation of organic bodies consist of the diverse and successive relations between movement and rest. Their quantity being determined, the number of possible relations between the one and the other must also be determined. The distance between two limits or points can be considered as representing the duration of life.

201. If one of these limits is movement and the other repose, the successive progression of the diverse proportions of one and of the other constitutes the march and revolution of life; beyond this point, we begin to die.

202. This progression of diverse modifications between movement and rest can be exactly proportioned, or this proportion can be disturbed.

203. If a man goes through this progression without this proportion being disturbed, he lives in perfect health and reaches his final days without illness. If these proportions are disturbed, illness ensues. Illness is therefore nothing more than a disturbance of the progression of the movement of life. This disturbance can be considered as existing in the solids or in the fluids. In the solids it upsets the harmony of the properties of organic parts, by diminishing some and

increasing others. In the fluids, it disturbs their local and internal movement. The aberration of movement in the solids—by changing their properties—disturbs the functions of the viscera, and therefore changes must result. The aberration of internal movement of the humors produces their degeneration. The aberration of local movement produces obstruction and fever: obstruction through the slackening or abolition of movement; fever through acceleration. Perfection of the solids or of the viscera consists of the harmony of all their properties and functions. The quality of the fluids, their internal and local movement, are the result of the functions of the viscera.

204. It is sufficient, therefore, in order to establish the general harmony of the body, to reestablish the functions of the viscera, because once their functions are reestablished, they assimilate everything which they can and separate what cannot be assimilated. This natural effort on the part of the viscera is called crisis.

Chapter 11: On Sickness

205. Sickness being the disturbance of harmony, this disturbance can be more or less considerable and produces effects more or less sensible; these effects are called *symptomatic symptoms*.

206. *Symptomatic symptoms* are effects produced by the cause of the malady. If, on the contrary, these effects are the efforts of nature to overcome the causes of the malady, to destroy such causes and to restore harmony, we call them *critical symptoms*.

207. In practice, it is important to distinguish between them carefully, in order to prevent or arrest the one and promote the other.

208. All the causes of illness more or less distort or derange

the proportions between matter and the movement of the viscera, and between the solids or fluids. Through their different applications, they produce a more or less marked abatement or perturbation within the properties of the matter and of the organs.

209. In order to remedy the effects of such abatement and perturbation, and in order to overcome them, one should therefore provoke the intension, that is, one must increase the irritability, *the elasticity, the fluidity, and the movement.*

210. A body which is in harmony is insensible to the effects of Magnetism, since the proportion of the established harmony cannot be changed by the application of a uniform and general action. On the other hand, a body which is in disharmony, that is, one in whose state the proportions are disturbed, in this state, whatever we have grown insensible to through habit becomes sensible through the application of Magnetism. This is so because the proportion of the dissonance is increased by such application.

211. Furthermore, we can understand also that as the illness approaches cure, one grows insensible to the Magnetism, and this is the *criterion* of cure.

212. We can also understand that the application of Magnetism frequently increases the suffering.

213. The action of Magnetism arrests the aberration of the state of harmony.

214. It is through the application of Magnetism that the symptoms cease.

215. Furthermore, it is also through Magnetism that the efforts of Nature against the causes of disease are increased, and consequently the critical symptoms are increased.

216. It is by these diverse effects that we succeed in distinguishing between the various symptoms.

217. The development of symptoms occurs in an inverse order to that by which the malady was formed.

218. We might represent the disease as a ball of twine which unwinds itself in the reverse order of which it began and by which it increased.

219. No illness can be cured without a crisis.

220. In a crisis one should observe three stages: perturbation, coction [literally "a cooking, or coming to the boiling point," (Ed.)], and evacuation.

Chapter 12: On Education

221. Man can be considered as existing either individually or as constituting a part of society: from these two points of view he can maintain universal harmony.

222. Among the animals, man is one of the species destined by nature to live in society.

223. The development of his faculties, the formation of his habits, under these two circumstances [i.e., individual or social life (Ed.)], produces what we call education.

224. The principle of education is therefore (1) The perfection of the primary faculties; (2) the harmonization of his habits with the universal harmony.

225. Man's education begins with his existence, that is, from the very moment the infant begins (1) to expose the organs of his senses to the impressions of external objects and (2) to deploy and exercise the movement of his limbs.

226. The perfection of the organs of sense consists (1) in irritability [i.e., the function of expansion and contraction of the body musculature, as described in the *Memoir of F. A. Mesmer, Doctor of Medicine, On His Discoveries, 1799,* (Ed.)] and (2) in all the possible combinations of their usage.

227. The perfection of the movement of his limbs consists in (1) their ease of operation, (2) their accuracy of direction, (3) their strength, (4) their equilibrium.

228. This development being a progression of life, the source of this development must be evaluated in the organization of each individual, the development being subject to the action of the universal influence, and of general and specific influences.

229. (1) The first rule, therefore, is to remove all obstacles which might disturb and impede that development.

230. (2) Successively placing the infant in an environment which will afford him the possibility of entire freedom to make all possible movements and trials.

231. Being uniquely obedient to the principle of nature which has formed his organs, the infant will find every single order which is compatible with his development, formation, and instruction.

232. Considered socially, man has two ways of being in communication with his fellow-creatures, through his ideas and his actions.

233. To communicate his ideas to other men, he has two means, either by natural or conventional language and writing.

234. Natural language is expressed in his physiognomy, voice, and gestures; natural writing is the faculty of being able to design anything which can speak to the eyes.

235. Conventional language consists of words; and conventional writing, of letters.

Chapter 13: Theory of Processes

236. It has been mentioned in the theory of the general system, that the universal currents were the cause of the existence of bodies, and that everything which was capable of accelerating these currents produced the intension or augmentation of the properties of these bodies. According to this principle, it is easy to conceive that if it was in our

power to accelerate these currents, we could, by increasing the energy of nature, extend at will the properties in all bodies and even restore those properties which some accident might have weakened. However, just as the water of a river cannot climb back toward its own source in order to increase the rapidity of its current, in the same way the constituent parts of the earth, subject to the laws of the universal currents, cannot act upon the original source of their existence. If we cannot act immediately upon the universal currents, can there not be a way, for all bodies in general, to act by particular means upon each other, in reciprocally accelerating among themselves the streams of the currents which transverse their interstices?

237. Just as there exists a general and reciprocal gravitation of all celestial bodies toward each other, so too does there exist a particular and reciprocal gravitation of the constituent parts of the earth towards the whole, and from this whole toward each part, and finally, from these parts toward each particular part. This mutual action of all bodies exerts itself by means of the currents ebbing and flowing, in a more or less direct manner, following the analogy of bodily forms. Therefore, of all the bodies, the one which can act most effectively upon man is his fellow-man. It is sufficient that a man be near another man in order to affect him, in order to provoke the intension of his properties.

238. The respective position of two beings who act, the one upon the other, is not a matter of indifference. To determine what this position should be, one should consider each being as a whole composed of diverse parts, each possessing a particular form and tonic movement. One may imagine, by this consideration, that the greatest possible influence of one upon the other occurs when they are so placed that their analogous parts act upon each other in the most exact opposition. In order for two men to act in the strongest possible

way, the one upon the other, they must be placed face to face. In this position they provoke the intension of their properties in a harmonic manner and can be considered as forming a whole. In an isolated individual, when a part of his body suffers, the entire life-action of his body directs itself toward that part, in order to overcome the cause of the suffering. Likewise, when two men act, the one upon the other, the entire action of this united effort is brought to bear upon the afflicted part, with a force proportionate to the increase of the mass. Thus, in general, one can say that the action of Magnetism increases by virtue of the masses. It is possible to direct the action of Magnetism more particularly upon an individual part. In order to do this, it is sufficient to establish a most exact continuity between the parts that are touched and the individual who touches. Our hands can be considered as proper *conductors* in establishing such continuity. It follows from what we have said regarding the most advantageous position of two beings acting the one upon the other that in order to maintain the harmony of the whole, we must touch the right side with the left hand and vice versa. It is from this necessity that the opposition of the poles of the human body results. These poles, as we observe in the magnet, are in opposition with regard to one another; they can be changed, communicated, destroyed, or reinforced.

239. To imagine the opposition of the poles, one should consider man as divided in two by a line drawn from top to bottom. All points of the left side can be considered as opposite poles to those of the corresponding points of the right side. Since the emission of the currents becomes more sensible through the extremities, we shall consider the extremities solely as poles in themselves. The left hand will be the pole opposed to the right hand, and so forth. Next, after considering the extremities as a whole, we can also

consider them from the point of view of opposing poles in each of them: thus, in the hand, the little finger will be the pole opposed to the thumb, the index finger will participate in the faculty of the thumb, and the third finger with that of the little finger; the action of the middle finger, being at the center of the equator of the magnet, will be deprived of any special property. The poles of the human body can be communicated to animate and inanimate bodies, the animate being more susceptible than the others, by virtue of their relative analogy with man and of the placement of their parts. It is sufficient to determine only one pole in any body in order immediately to establish the opposite pole. One can destroy this determination by touching the same body in the reverse way from which one has touched it initially, and one can reinforce the pole already established by touching the opposite pole with the other hand.
240. The action of Animal Magnetism can be reinforced and propagated through animate and inanimate bodies. Just as this action increases by virtue of masses, the more one adds magnetic bodies one to the other so that the poles are not contrary, that is to say, so that they touch each other at opposite poles, the more will one reinforce the action of Magnetism. The bodies most suitable for reinforcing and propagating Animal Magnetism are animate bodies; then comes vegetable matter; and in those classes of substance without life, iron and glass act with the most intensity.

Chapter 14: Observations on Nervous Diseases

241. The exaggerated irritability of the nerves produced by the aberration of harmony within the human body is what we designate, more particularly, *nervous diseases*.
242. There are as many varieties of these diseases as there are variations among all the possible numbers of combinations that one can suppose.

243. (1) The general irritability can be increased or diminished through an infinity of nuances.

244. (2) Different organs may be particularly affected, while others may not.

245. (3) One can conceive of an infinite number of connections, resulting by varying degrees, in which each of the organs may be individually affected.

246. A careful and attentive observer will find a wealth of instruction in the numberless phenomena which produce nervous maladies. It is in these conditions that one can most easily study the properties and the faculties of the human body.

247. Also, it is in these conditions that one can convince oneself, through the observation of facts, how we are dependent upon the action of all the creatures which surround us, and how any change in these beings or in their relationship to each other can never be absolutely indifferent to us

248. The extension of the properties and faculties of our organs, being considerably increased in these types of maladies, should enable us also to extend the limit of our knowledge, in enabling us to understand a multitude of impressions about which we would otherwise have no idea.

249. In order to understand and fully appreciate all that I have said, one should keep in mind the mechanisms of sensations attendant upon my principles.

250. The faculty of perceiving impressions is the result, in man, of two principal conditions, the one external, the other internal. The first is the degree of intensity with which an external object acts upon our organs; the second is the degree of susceptibility with which the organ receives the action of an external object.

251. [I have taken the liberty of revising the "literal" meaning of this aphorism, and, for the sake of clarity, render it

as follows (Ed.).] If the action of an external object is three-dimensional, and the particular organ for which such action is destined is capable of perceiving it only as two-dimensional, then it is clear that I may never have any knowledge of the reality of such objects. However, if through whatever means, I could succeed in rendering my organ capable of perceiving three-dimensional action, or I am able to determine that such objects naturally act in three dimensions, in either of these cases, the reality of these objects will become known to me.

252. Until now, human intelligence has not dreamed of increasing the external scope of our senses by increasing the condition of sensations, that is, by increasing the *internality* of the action which these senses exert upon us. Through the invention of glasses, microscopes and telescopes, the extension of a sense has been accomplished for sight. By this means we have pierced the darkness which concealed from us an entire universe, infinitely small and infinitely large.

253. How much has philosophy not profitted by such ingenious discovery? Have not absurdities been demonstrated in ancient systems, concerning the nature of bodies? And what new truths cannot be perceived by the attentive eye of an observer?

254. Of what avail would have been the genius of Descartes, Galileo, Newton, Kepler, Buffon, without the extension of the organ of sight? Perhaps great things; but astronomy and natural history would still be at the point where they were found by these men.

255. If the extension of one sense has been able to produce a considerable revolution in our knowledge, what still vaster field has again opened itself to our observation, if, as I believe, the extension of the faculties of each sense, of each organ, can be carried as far and even farther than lenses

have carried the extension of sight; if this extension can succeed in enabling us to appreciate a multitude of impressions which would remain unknown to us, of comparing these impressions, of combining them, and thus gaining an intimate and particular knowledge of the objects which produce them, of the forms of these objects, their properties, the relationships between them, and even of the particles of which they are comprised.

256. In ordinary usage, we can only judge anything through the cooperation of the combined impressions of all our senses. One might say that we are, through the rapport with the objects which the extension of a sense has enabled us to perceive, like an individual deprived of all his senses except sight would be in regard to everything which surrounds us. Certainly, if a creature so deprived could exist, the scope of his knowledge would be severely restricted; and we can consider that he would not have the same idea of objects more sensible to us.

257. Let us suppose that we restore to this physically handicapped creature, successively, each of the senses which he does not have. What a multitude of discoveries would he not make instantly! Each impression which the same object produced upon another of his organs would furnish him with a new idea of that object. It would be very difficult for him to understand how these diverse ideas pertained to the same object. It would be necessary beforehand that he combine them, that he verify the results by a number of experiences. In the infancy of his faculties, this man would perhaps need more than a month to be able to appreciate what a bottle is, or a chandelier, etc., in order that he have the same ideas that we have concerning them.

258. All of the slight impressions by which objects in our environment affect us, through our contact with them in our normal condition, make themselves known to us in

various ways. Such ways and such contact are not available in the case of the man just referred to. The properties of our organs, in the necessary harmony that constitutes human beings, have only a certain degree of extension for each of them, beyond which we are not able to perceive anything.

259. But when, through a *loss* of the faculties in any parts, the properties of another organ reach a certain point of extension, we then become susceptible to appreciating and knowing impressions which were entirely unknown to us before. This is what we find at any moment in observing individuals afflicted with nervous disorders.

260. The quality of impressions of which they have knowledge thereby is absolutely new to them. At first they are astonished, frightened. But soon, through habit, they become familiar with them and in time succeed in availing themselves of their utility, just as we avail ourselves of knowledge which experience brings us in a state of sanity. Thus it is a mistake for us to ascribe to fantasies all the peculiarities which we observe in the behavior of these individuals. What motivates and determines their actions is as real a cause as those which determine the actions of more rational men. There exists a difference only in the motivation of these creatures, which renders them sensible to a multitude of impressions of which we are unaware.

261. What is unfortunate for the convenience of our instruction is that these persons subject to crises lose nearly all recollection of their impressions upon returning to their ordinary state. If it were not for this, if they maintained their conceptions completely, they themselves could bring to us all the observations I have suggested to you, with more facility than I can express. But what these persons cannot relate to us in their ordinary state, can we not learn from them when they are in a state of crisis? If these are true sensations which motivate them, they should, when they

are in a condition to appraise and consider them, be able
to render an account just as exact as we would be able to
give each other of all objects which actually affect us.

262. I realize that what I am advancing must appear exaggerated and impossible to those whose circumstances
have not enabled them to make these observations, but I
entreat them to suspend their judgment. It is not upon one
fact alone that I base my opinion. The uniqueness of these
facts has induced me to add proof upon proof, in order to
assure myself of their reality.

263. I therefore believe that it is possible, in studying nervous persons subject to crises, to make them render an exact
account of sensations which they experience. I further state
that, with care and persistence, one can, by exercising in
them this faculty of explaining what they perceive, and by
perfecting their manner of appreciating these new sensations, so to speak, further their education for this condition.
It is gratifying to work with patients so trained, in order to
instruct oneself in all the phenomena which result from the
exaggerated irritability of the senses. Moreover, after awhile,
the time comes when the attentive observer himself becomes susceptible to appreciating whatever sensations these
individuals experience, by the frequently repeated compari-
sons between his own impressions with those of the person
in crisis. The use of this faculty, which is in all of us, can
be considered as a truly difficult art, but one which is,
nevertheless, possible to acquire, like others, through study
and application.

264. I could speak in more detail at another time. Let us
discuss the diverse phenomena which I have observed in
persons in crisis. Anyone may verify them when he finds
himself in circumstances similar to those in which I have
been placed.

265. In nervous maladies, when in a state of crisis, irritability

upon the retina advances to a greater degree, and the eye becomes capable of perceiving microscopic objects. All that the art of the Optician has been able to imagine cannot even approach to that degree of perception. In the most obscure darkness there is still preserved enough light for these subjects to see by and gather a sufficient quantity of rays, in order to distinguish the shapes of different objects, and determine their relationships. They can also determine objects through bodies which appear opaque to us, which proves that the opacity in bodies is not only a particular quality but also a circumstance relative to the degree of irritability of our organs.

266. One patient that I have treated, and several others whom I have carefully observed, have furnished me with a number of experiences in that regard.

267. One of them perceived the pores of the skin as a considerable size. She described the structure in conformity with what the microscope has taught us. But she went further. The skin appeared as a sieve to her. Through it she saw the texture of the muscles, all at the correct locations, and the junction of bones in passages devoid of pulp. All this she explained in an ingenious kind of way, and sometimes she was impatient at the sterility and insufficiency of our expressions for communicating her ideas. A very thin opaque body did not prevent her from distinguishing objects, but only sensibly diminished the impressions which she received, as would a glass to us.

268. For such reasons, therefore, she can see even better than I, and with her eyelids closed. Many times when she was in that state, in order to verify the truth of what she told me, I placed her hand upon different objects, and she was never deceived.

269. It is this same person who, in complete darkness, perceived all the poles of the human body clearly, as a luminous

vapor; not that it was like fire, but the impression which it made upon her organs gave her an idea akin to fire, which she could express only by the word *light*.

270. I observed that one should consider what she stated concerning a variety of her perceptions as being due to the particular impression that these poles made upon her organ of sight, and not as any final idea which one should grasp.

271. It is in that state that it is infinitely interesting to verify all the principles which I have given in my theory of the poles of the body.

272. Had I known nothing [of these phenomena (Ed.)], and by the merest chance had attempted this experience, this patient would have instructed me.

273. On my face she perceived my eyes and nose. The luminous rays which emanated from the eyes proceeded to join with the rays from the nose, reinforcing them. From there, they were directed toward the nearest point that one opposed to them. However, if I wished to observe objects off to one side, without turning my head, then the rays from the eyes separated from the end of my nose, in order to proceed in the direction that I wished them to go.

274. Each tip of the eyelashes, eyebrows, and hairs give a feeble light. The neck appears slightly luminous, the chest dimly lighted. If I present my hands to her, immediately the thumb becomes distinguished by a vivid light, the little finger being half as much, the index and third fingers seem lighted by only a borrowed light. The middle finger is obscure. The palm of the hand is also luminous.

275. If the exaggerated irritability proceeds to other organs, they become the same as sight, sensitive to perceiving the slightest impressions analogous to their constitution, of which they were totally ignorant beforehand.

276. There is a vast field of observation which is open to us, but it is very difficult to recount. Here art abandons us.

It cannot furnish us such means as to verify by comparison what is taught to us by persons in crisis.

277. We have only the poorest type of microscopic device for hearing; we have no type [of microscopic device (Ed.)] for odor or touch, and further, we have no practice in appreciating results proven by comparatively perfected senses, results which can be varied to infinity.

278. But if art abandons us, nature remains with us. She is sufficient for us. Although the infant who enters the world with all his organs is unaware of their resources, nevertheless, nature shows him their usage in the successive development of his faculties. This education takes place without system; it is submissive to circumstances. The instruction that I propose should be accomplished in the same way— that is, to renounce all kinds of routine which fail to lend themselves to simple observations that circumstances furnish. At first you will only perceive an immense pool. You will not be able to distinguish anything. But little by little the dawn will break for you, and the sphere of your knowledge will be increased at the same time as your perception of objects.

279. Frequently persons in crisis are tormented by a noise which stuns them, which they can discern, and which they characterize in a very real way. Without approaching any closer to the source of that noise, you may be able to become aware of it.

280. Many times I have observed a person affected with nervous maladies who could not listen to the sound of a horn without falling into the strongest crisis. Frequently I have observed her complain that she heard one, and finish by falling into very strong convulsions, saying that it was approaching her. And it was only after upwards of a quarter of an hour that I was able to hear it.

281. We will observe the same phenomena for taste. Of twenty foods that we diluted to an extreme degree, a person

in crisis, in whom irritability was considerably increased on the tongue and palate, could perceive a variety of taste and flavors in these foods.

282. I know a very spiritual person whose nerves are extremely irritable, who, having this irritation uniquely on the tongue, and maintaining her judgment, has told me many times: "In eating this small piece of bread, as large as the head of a pin, it seems to me that I have a considerable mouthful, of an exquisite flavor. But what is quite singular is the fact that not only do I sense the flavor of a fine morsel of bread, but also I sense separately the taste of all the particles which compose it: the water, the farina, all finally produce upon me a multitude of sensations that I cannot express, and which give me ideas that succeed each other with extreme rapidity, but which cannot be appreciated in words."

283. The sense of smell is also able to become more sensitive by as great an extension of faculty as is taste. I have observed patients distinguish the slightest odors at very great distances, and even through closed doors. At other times, some persons to whom odor is so sensible distinguish the diverse original odors that the Perfumer has employed in compounding a perfume.

284. But of all the senses, the one which presents us with the most phenomena for observation is that which we have had least knowledge about, up to the present: touch.

Chapter 15: Processes of Animal Magnetism

285. We have seen from my Doctrine that everything in the universe is contiguous by means of a universal fluid in which all bodies are immersed.

286. There is a continuous circulation which establishes the necessity of currents coming and going.

287. There are many ways to establish and strengthen them upon man. The surest way is to place oneself in opposition to the person one wishes to touch, that is, face to face, so that one presents his right side to the left side of the patient. In order to establish harmony with him, one must first place his hands upon the patient's shoulders, then proceed along the length of the arms as far as the tips of the fingers, holding the thumbs of the patient for a moment; then recommencing two or three times, after which one establishes the currents from the head to the feet. One searches out the cause and site of the illness and pain; but more often it is by touch and reasoning that you may assure yourself of the seat and the cause of the malady and pain, which in the majority of illnesses resides in the side opposite to the pain, especially in paralyses, rheumatism, and other illnesses of this type.

288. Having fully assured yourself of this preliminary procedure, you constantly touch the cause of the malady, maintaining the symptomatic pains, until you have rendered them critical. In this way you assist nature's effort against the cause of the malady, and you occasion a salutary crisis, which is the sole means of curing radically. You assuage the pains which we call symptomatic symptoms, which yield to the touch, without as yet acting upon the cause of the malady (that which we distinguish by the name *symptomatics*), which pains, being initially irritated by touch, are terminated by a crisis, after which the malady becomes relieved and the cause of the malady diminished.

289. The seat of almost all maladies is ordinarily in the viscera of the lower belly; the stomach, spleen, liver, the omentum, mesentery, kidneys, etc. The cause of all maladies or aberrations is an engorgement, obstruction, disturbance or suppression of circulation in a part, which, compressing the blood vessels or lymphatics, and especially the nerve branches, more or less considerably, occasions a spasm

or a tension within the parts wherein they lead, especially in those parts in which the fibers have less natural elasticity, as in the brain, lungs, etc., or in those parts where fluid circulates sluggishly and thickly, like the synovia, destined to facilitate movement and articulation. If these engorgements compress a nerve trunk or a considerable part of a branch, the movement and sensibility of the parts to which it corresponds is entirely suppressed, as in apoplexy, paralysis, etc.

290. In addition to the primary reason for touching the viscera first (that is, in order to discover the cause of the malady), there is one other more determining reason: The nerves are the best conductors of Magnetism which exist in the body. The nerves are in so great a number within the viscera that many physicians have placed there the seat of the sensations of the soul. Most abundant and sensible are the nervous center of the diaphragm, the solar plexus, umbilical, etc. This mass of an infinity of nerves corresponds with all parts of the body.

291. One touches, in the position previously indicated, with the thumb and the index finger, or with the palm of the hand, or with one finger reinforced solely by the other, by describing a line on the part that we wish to touch, and in following, as closely as possible, the direction of the nerves. One touches also with all five fingers open and slightly curved. Touching at a short distance from the part is stronger, because a current exists between the hand or the conductor and the patient.

292. One can touch indirectly with advantage by using a foreign conductor. Most commonly we can use a short rod about ten to fifteen inches long [actually "thumbs," (Ed.)], cone-shaped, and terminated by a truncated point. The base of this conductor is about three, five, or six lines in width. [A *ligne* might possibly be one-twelfth of an inch, this being

an obsolete medical definition of a "line." (Ed.).] The point is from one to two [lines wide]. After glass, which is the best conductor, we can use iron, steel, gold, silver, etc., preferring the denser body, because the channels of such bodies are narrower and more multiplied. They have an action proportionate to the smaller diameter of the interstices. If the rod is magnetized its action is greater. However, you should determine from the circumstances what is to be used, as in the case of inflammation of the eyes, for example, or too great erethism, etc., in which it would be harmful. It is therefore wise to have two conductors [one magnetized, the other not (Ed.)]. We magnetize with a cane or some other foreign conductor by paying attention to the fact that by using such a foreign body the polarity is changed, and that we touch differently with a conductor, that is, from right to right, and from left to left.

293. It is also good to oppose one pole to the other. That is, if one touches the head, the chest, the stomach, etc., with the right hand, he should oppose the left hand from the posterior part, chiefly along the line which separates the body in two parts, that is, from the center of the forehead to the pubis, because, the body representing a magnet, once you establish the north to the right side, the left side becomes the south, and the midline is the equator, which is without any predominant action. In such opposition of one hand to the other, you establish the poles.

294. One reinforces the action of Magnetism by multiplying the currents upon the patient. There are many more advantages to touching face to face than any other way: because the currents emanating from your viscera and from all the extensions of the body establish a circulation with the patient. The same basis proves the usefulness of trees, ropes, irons and chains, etc.

295. A basin and bath become magnetized in the same

manner, by plunging the cane or some other conductor into the water, in order to establish a current within it. By agitating the water in a straight line, the person placed in opposition to it will feel the effect of it. If the basin is large, we establish four points, which become the four cardinal points, by tracing a line in the water along the side of the basin, from the east to the north, thence from the west and the south to the north. Many persons can be placed around this basin, and there they can experience the Magnetic effects. If there are a great number of persons, we can trace many radii leading to each of them, after acting upon the mass of water as much as possible.

296. A baquet [tub] is a kind of rounded or oval-shaped quadrangle, of a diameter proportionate to the number of patients that we wish to treat. It is made from stout staves, assembled, painted and joined so that it can contain water, to a depth of approximately one foot, the upper part wider than the base by three to six inches, enclosed by a two-piece cover, which is mounted upon the tank and fixed there by large nails. Inside the baquet you arrange bottles like radii converging from the circumference to the center . . . all of the same height, having left a space between them sufficient to receive the neck of another. After this, you set one bottle in the midst of the vessel, vertically or horizontally, from which emanate all the radii that you first made with some small bottles, followed by larger ones, when the divergence permits. The bottom of the first is at the center, its neck inserted into the base of the succeeding one, so that the neck of the last ends at the circumference of the baquet. These bottles should be filled with water, corked and magnetized in the same way; it is desirable that this be done by the same person. To give greater strength to the baquet we can add a second and even a third layer of bottles atop

the first. Usually, we make a second row which starts at the center and covers the first row to the half or three-quarter mark. We then add water to the tank sufficient to cover all the bottles. We can add thereto iron filings, crushed glass, and similar things, about which I have expressed different opinions.

297. We can also make a baquet without water, by filling the spaces between the bottles with crushed glass, iron filings, and sand. Whether we use water or the other materials, we indicate on the cover the points at which the holes are to be made to receive the iron rods which lead into the baquet (at a distance from eight to ten inches from its walls) between the bottoms of the bottles in the first row. The iron rods are of a flexible type which enter in a straight line to the bottom of the baquet and curve out from the holes. The rods are constructed so that, ending in obtuse points, they can be used in touching parts of the body, such as the forehead, eye, ear, stomach, etc., etc.

298. From the interior or exterior of the baquet, individually, an ample cord is attached to an iron rod. The patient can apply this cord to the suffering part. Holding this cord, patients can form a chain, and placing the left thumb upon their neighbor's right, or the right upon the left, so that the insides of the thumbs touch, they draw as near to each other as they possibly can. They establish contact with one another at the thighs, knees, and feet, and form, so to speak, a contiguous body, through which the magnetic fluid circulates continually and is reinforced by all the different points of contact, to which may also be added the position of two patients who face each other. We also have some rods long enough to reach those of the second row, through spaces between those in the first.

299. We can make small individual baquets, called mag-

netic boxes, for the use of patients who cannot go for treatment, or who, because of the nature of their illness, have need of continuous treatment. These boxes can be composed more or less: the simplest type contains only a bottle, placed horizontally and filled with water or ground glass, enclosed within a box, from whence comes a rod or a cord. A single bottle alone, applied on a part, might even prove more effective. One can employ many of them in a layer and containing some iron mixed in the neck of each, which can produce a sensible effect. The commonest type are boxes of about a foot in width, height and length proportionate to what they are to contain. The height should not ordinarily exceed that of the bed, which is about ten to twelve inches. Within the box we placed four or more bottles, as we wish, prepared and arranged like those of the baquet. If the box is designed to be used upon a bed, we take some smaller bottles, half of which are filled with water and the others with glass. Those filled with water are corked; those which are filled with glass are armed with a small conductor of iron, which is sealed in the neck of those bottles, projecting from the cover of the box. The spaces between bottles are filled with ground glass, either dry or moistened. A cord wound around the neck of each bottle extends through a hole in the side of the box and communicates all bottles to each other. The cover is grooved and fastened by a screw. We place this box upon the bed, and the cords, extending from the right and the left sides, are placed upon the bed or between the sheets or upon the covers, extending to the patient.

300. The bottles to be used that day are filled with water or glass, prepared, and placed as in the large baquet. We can then add a cord and some rods and convert it to a family baquet.

301. The denser the material which fills these bottles, the greater is the action. If we could fill them with mercury they would possess the most action.

302. There are many ways to increase the number and the activity of the currents. If you wish to touch a patient with force, gather together as many people as possible in his apartment. Establish a chain of people which leads from the patient and ends at the magnetiser. One person leaning against the magnetiser, or with his hand upon his shoulder, increases his action. There is an infinity of additional ways I might relate, such as using sound, music, light, mirrors, etc.

303. The magnetic current maintains its effect for some time after having left the body, in much the same way as the sound from a flute diminishes in retiring. Magnetism at a certain distance produces a greater effect than when it is applied immediately.

304. After man and animals, plants and especially trees are the most susceptible to Animal Magnetism. In order to magnetize a tree beneath which you desire to establish a treatment, choose a young one, vigorous, with branches, and insofar as it is possible, one with straight fibers and without knots. Although all types of trees may serve, the denser ones, such as the oak, the elm, are more susceptible. Having made your selection, you place yourself at a certain distance from the south side, establish a right and a left side, which form the two poles, and the line of demarcation at the center, the equator. With a finger, the iron rod, or a cane, follow along the leaves, the ramifications, and the branches. After having conducted many of these lines to a main branch, you conduct the currents to the trunk, down to the roots. Begin again until you have magnetized the entire side, then you magnitize the other side in the same manner and with the same hand, because the currents coming

from the conductor are diverged within it. They come together again at a certain distance and are not subject to
repulsion. The north is magnetized through the same procedure. This operation completed, you approach the tree,
and, after having magnetized any visible roots, you embrace
the tree, presenting all your poles thereto. The tree possesses then all the virtues of Magnetism. Healthy people
who rest upon the tree at any time thereafter, or touch it,
can experience its effect. And sick people, especially those
already magnetized, experience its effects violently and will
undergo crises. In order to establish treatment there, attach
cords, at a certain height, to the trunk and to the main
branches, numerous and long, more or less in proportion to
the persons who are gathered there and who, facing the
tree and placed circularly, either seated or on mats, are
positioned according to their afflicted parts, just as they are
at the baquet. They are encircled [presumably by the cord
(Ed.)] as often as possible and experience crises as they
would at the baquet, but in a milder form. The tree's curative
effect is much more prompt and more active in proportion
to the number of patients, who increase the energy of it by
multiplying the currents, the force, and the contacts. The
wind shaking the branches of the tree adds to its action.
It is similar in action to a stream or a waterfall, if one is
fortunate enough to have one available at the spot which
is chosen. If many trees are near one another, we can magnetize them and join them by cords, from one to the other.
The patients detect an indefinable odor from the trees, which
is very disagreeable to them and which remains with them
for some time after having left the trees, and which they
resent upon returning. We cannot be certain as to the length
of time a tree maintains the Magnetism. We believe that
it may last for many months. To be sure, however, renew
it from time to time.

305. In order to magnetize a bottle, hold it by its two ends, which you rub with your fingers, stroking towards both ends. You separate the hand successively from the extremity, as you compress, so to speak, the fluid. You hold a glass or a vase in the same manner, and you magnetize the fluid which it contains. taking care when you offer it to the patient who is going to drink it that you hold it between the thumb and the little finger, allowing him to drink from it in this manner. The patient experiences a taste which would not exist had the fluid been drunk in a different way.

306. A flower of whatever kind is magnetized by touching it with principle and intension.

307. In rubbing the two ends of a bathtub with the fingers, rod or cane, they descend to the water whereupon one describes a line, in the same direction and repeated many times —thus do we magnetize a bath. Also, we can agitate the water in different ways, by insisting always on the line described, in which the great current reunites the smaller currents adjoining it and is reinforced by them. If the patient within the bath finds the water too cold, we plunge a cane into it, and we direct a current therein by stroking it. This action is experienced by the patient as a sensation of warmth, which he attributes to the water. In places where there is a baquet or trees, we conduct a cord which can take the place of all other preparations. If we cannot magnetize, I believe that many bottles filled with magnetized water, and placed in the bath along the direction of the body, should produce the same effect. A little salt water added to the bath increases its tonicity.

308. In the center of the baquet one should place a glass vase, either cylindrical or of similar shape, which would have an opening in the top suitable for receiving a conductor, which, being fastened to the base of the vase in funnel or finger-like form, emanates from the baquet. The vase itself

should be pierced by lateral holes, through which the rods from the bottles are transmitted. The conductor could also be of glass.

Chapter 16: General Considerations on the Magnetic Treatment

309. There is only one illness and one cure. Perfect harmony of all our organs and their functions constitutes health. Illness is only the aberration of this harmony. Therefore, cure consists in reestablishing the harmony that has been disturbed. The general remedy is the application of Magnetism by the designated means. Movement can be increased or diminished in a body; movement must moderate or excite it. It is upon the solids that the effect of Magnetism is induced, the action of the viscera being the means by which nature helps herself in order to prepare, separate, or assimilate the humors. These are the functions of the organs that must be rectified. Without entirely proscribing any remedies, either internal or external, one must nevertheless use them with great care, because they can be contraindicated, or useless: contraindicated when they act, for the most part, too harshly, thereby increasing the irritation, spasm, or other effects that are contrary to harmony, which it is necessary to reestablish and maintain. Such are the violent purgatives, hot diuretics, aperitives, the blistering agents, and all the epispastics —useless, because such remedies, received into the stomach and liver, receive the same action as food. Thus the parts analogous to our humors are assimilated, while the heterogeneous elements are expelled through the excretions.

310. Magnetic fluid does not act upon alien bodies, nor upon those which are outside of the vascular system; when the stomach contains putridity, pollution, or an over-abundance of bile, one has recourse to emetics or purgatives.

311. If acidity dominates or prevails, one administers absorbants such as magnesia; (1) if it is alkaline, one prefers acids, such as cream of tartar; (2) if we wish to administer purgatives, they should be given in the dose of one or two ounces. A smaller dose becomes a thirst producer, suitable for neutralizing the acid or alkali, and establishing evacuation thereby. Since the alkali dominates more often than acidity, we ordinarily prescribe an acid regimen: salad, currants, gooseberries, cherries, lemonade, acid syrups, etc.

312. Decrease in movement and of vigor being the result of the greater part of illness, not only must we direct the diet, but also we urge the patient to partake of nourishment. According to the methods which I have just mentioned, those foods which are desired by patients should be allowed them. It is rare that nature misleads them.

313. Strong wine, liqueurs, coffee, very spicy foods, by themselves or their ingredients, are prohibited. Tobacco is also prohibited, because its irritating effect is propagated by the pituitary membrane, within the throat, chest, head, and occasions contractions contrary to harmony. The usual drink is good wine diluted with much water that is pure or acidulated. Washing and baths are very helpful. We use bloodletting in inflammation or in inflammatory disposition, or in genuine or false plethora.

314. Since it is not my intention to give a general history of illnesses and of their treatment, we will cite only those which offer themselves most often to treatment by Magnetism, and the manner of applying it, according to observations made, especially in the treatment of M. le Marquis de Tissard à Beaubourg.

315. In epilepsy, we touch the head, be it on the top, or at the base of the nose with one hand, and the knuckles of the other. In the viscera, we seek the principal causes which usually converge there. By our double touching we break

down obstructions in the viscera, and the engorgement, which in the epileptic is situated within the brain (upon which we began), and thus activate almost all the nerves of the system. Catalepsy is treated in the same manner.

316. In apoplexy our touching proceeds upon the main organs, such as the breast, stomach, especially at the site we call the pit (below the xiphoid cartilage), the site of the nervous center of the diaphragm, which reunites an infinity of nerves. We also touch, by opposition, the spinal column, tracing it to the large intercostal muscles, which are situated an inch or two from the spine, from the neck to the base of the trunk. We must persist until we obtain crisis, and gather all possible means of intensifying the Magnetism, either by the iron rod or the chain (of human beings), which you form with as many persons as you can assemble. Once the patient has been restored to a condition wherein his impressions are normal, and the crisis having been obtained, the situation in regard to any initial results and the cause of the malady will indicate to you what is suitable to undertake and whether evacuants should be employed.

317. In diseases of the ear, the patient places the cord around his head, one rod from the baquet in his ear and one in his mouth. In cases of deafness, as in paralysis where speech is impeded, and with mutes, touching is done by placing the thumbs in the ear, spreading the other fingers, and presenting them to the currents of the magnetic fluid, or by gathering the currents at a distance and bringing them back with the palm of the hand to the head, where we apply the hand for some time.

318. Illnesses of the eyes are treated with the iron rod or the end of the fingers, which we present to the part, and which we use in stroking the eyeball and eyelid. We also use the rod especially in cases of cataract. In case inflammation exists, one should touch with extreme lightness.

319. Tinea is touched directly, bathing it morning and evening with magnetized water, the cord to the head.

320. Tumors of all kinds, lymphatic and sanguine engorgements, sores, and even ulcers experience excellent results. Lotions with magnetized water, local baths with such water, either cold or tepid, and the usual treatment, bring about astonishing results. Patients suffering from vivid pains in ulcerated or injured parts, are quickly relieved by encircling them with the cord.

321. By these few details, it is evident that Magnetism is useful in cutaneous and internal maladies.

322. Disorders of the head are touched on the front, the top, at the parietals, the frontal sinus, and the brow; on the stomach and other viscera which contain the cause.

323. Disorders of the teeth are treated by touching upon the articulations of the jaws and related parts.

324. Leprosy is treated like tinea, placing the cord to the affected parts.

325. In speech difficulties, or the total negation occasioned chiefly through paralysis, we magnetize the mouth with the iron rod, and the exterior of the motor muscles of this organ by touching them.

326. The same methods are employed in disorders of the neck, chiefly at the lymphatics. Also, we magnetize the pituitary membrane, so that it likewise is joined to the other parts in treatment, and to the affects of those parts which are spread to the chest.

327. In migraine headaches we touch the stomach and temporal regions, where the pain is felt.

328. Asthma, oppression, and other affections of the chest are touched on such parts, by slowly passing one hand over the front of the chest and the other along the spine, allowing them to remain for a time upon the upper part, and descend-

ing slowly to the stomach, whereupon the hand is allowed
to remain also, especially in humid asthma.

329. The patient with nightmares is treated in the same manner, instructing him not to lie upon his back until he is cured.

330. Pain, engorgements, obstructions of the stomach, liver,
spleen, and the other viscera, are touched locally, and require more or less time and perserverance, in proportion to
the volume, age, and hardness of the tumors.

331. In colic, vomiting, nervous irritability, and intestinal
pain, as well as pain in the lower abdomen, we touch the
source of pain very lightly. In cases where inflammation
exists, or an inflammatory disposition, in such circumstances
we must avoid frictional touching of any kind.

332. In disorders of the womb, one touches not only the
viscera but also the breasts, the ovaries, and the large ligaments which are situated in the lateral and posterior parts,
and the round parts of the groin. In accordance with these
observances, the palm of the hand applied to the vulva expedites the menstrual flow and remedies leakages; this application is beneficial also in cases of dropping of the womb
and slackening of the muscles of the vagina.

Chapter 17: Concerning Crisis

333. A disease cannot be cured without a crisis. The crisis
is an effort of nature against the disease, tending, by an increase of movement, tone, and intension, through the action
of the magnetic fluid, to disperse the obstacles which impede
circulation, to dissolve and evacuate the molecules which
form such obstructions, and to reestablish harmony and equilibrium within all parts of the body.

334. Crises can be more or less evident, more or less salutary,
natural, or provoked.

335. Natural crises should be attributed only to the natural

constitution, which acts effectively upon the cause of the malady and which rids the body of such causes by different excretions, as in fevers, wherein the natural constitution alone triumphs over that which is harmful to it and expels it by spontaneous vomiting, movement of the bowels, sweating, urinating, hemorrhagic flow, etc.

336. The less evident crises are those in which the natural constitution acts insensibly, without violence, by slowly breaking down the obstacles which constrict the circulation, and drives them away through insensible processes.

337. When the natural constitution is insufficient to establish crises, we aid it through Magnetism, which, being put into action by the means indicated, in conjunction with the natural constitution, brings about the desired revolution. It is beneficial when, after having experienced a crisis, the patient feels comfortable and relieved, and principally when it is followed by advantageous evacuations.

338. The baquet, the iron rod, the cord and the chain contribute to crises. If such crises are judged too weak to act victoriously upon the malady, we increase them by touching the site of the pain and the cause. When we decide that the crisis has reached its limit, which is announced by a calm, we allow it to terminate itself. Or, when we believe it to be sufficient, we retire the patient to the state of sleep and insensibility, in which he is rested.

339. It is rare that a natural crisis is not salutary.

340. The one and the other often throw the patient into a cataleptic state, which should not frighten you and which terminates itself with the crisis.

341. In the case of erethism, of irritability, and of excessive susceptibility to such, it is dangerous to provoke and maintain unduly strong crises, because we thereby increase the disorder which these dispositions proclaim in the animal economy. Thus we would contribute to the intension of such

dispositions, when we should bring about remission; we increase the tendency to inflammation, we suspend, we suppress the evacuations which should bring about the cure, and we are diametrically in opposition to the purpose and efforts of nature.

342. When we excite violent crises in a subject who is disposed to them, we maintain in the organs a condition of forced elasticity which diminishes in the fiber the faculty of reacting to itself and of acting upon the humors which such fiber contains. From this there follows a kind of inertia, which maintains the condition against nature which we brought about. Such an habitual state is opposed to all efforts of nature against the cause of the malady. It increases the aberration and causes a wrinkle or fold to form within the organs, similar to a crease in material, which is very difficult to efface.

343. We observe on the one hand the advantage and necessity of crises; and on the other hand, the misuse which we can make of them.

344. A physician who is schooled in the doctrine of Animal Magnetism and who is an accurate observer of the effects of crises, will be able to derive from them all the benefits which they afford and will guard himself against the dangers of their abuse.

Bibliography

1. Anderson, Emily. *Mozart's Letters to His Family* (3 vols.). London: Macmillan and Co., 1938.
2. Bruce, William C. *Benjamin Franklin Self-Revealed* (2 vols.). New York: G. P. Putnam's Sons, 1917.
3. Carlyle, Thomas. *The French Revolution* (2 vols.). New York and London: The Colonial Press, 1900.
4. Ciba Symposia. *Mesmerism*. Vol. 9, no. 11, Mar.-Apr. 1948. Ciba Pharmaceutical Products, Inc. Summit, N. J.
5. Dakin, Edwin F. *Mrs. Eddy*. New York: Grosset & Dunlap, 1929.
6. du Commun, Dr. Joseph. *Three Lectures on Animal Magnetism*. New York, 1829.
7. Eden, Jerome. *Orgone Energy—The Answer to Atomic Suicide*. New York: Exposition Press, 1972.
8. Esdaile, James, M.D. *Mesmerism in India*, 1850. (Reissued by Julian Press, New York, 1957, as *Hypnosis in Medicine and Surgery*.)
9. Franklin, Benjamin. *Report of Dr. Benjamin Franklin and Other Commissioners*. London, 1785.
10. Galdston, Iago. *Progress in Medicine*. New York: Knopf, 1940.
11. Goldsmith, Margaret. *Franz Anton Mesmer*. London, 1934.
12. Goodman, Nathan G., ed. *The Ingenious Dr. Franklin*. Philadelphia: University of Pennsylvania Press, 1931.
13. Hall, Charles R., M.D. *Mesmerism—Its Rise, Progress and Mysteries*. New York, 1845.
14. Ince, Richard Basil. *Franz Anton Mesmer*. London: William Rider & Son, Ltd., 1920.
15. *Journal of Orgonomy*. Box 565, Ansonia Station, New York, N. Y. 10023.
16. Johnson, Charles P. *A Treatise on Animal Magnetism*. New York: Burgess & Stringer, 1844.
17. Lang, William. *Mesmerism—Its History, Phenomena and Practice*. Edinburgh: Fraser & Co., 1843.
18. Mesmer, Anton. *Mesmerism*. With an introduction by Gilbert Frankau. London: Macdonald, 1948. (This is Mesmer's *Memoir of 1779*.)

217

19. Parson, Frederick. *Vital Magnetism—Its Power Over Disease.* New York: Adams Victor & Co., 1877.
20. Reich, Wilhelm. *The Discovery of the Orgone.* Vol. 1, *The Function of the Orgasm.* New York: Orgone Institute Press, 1948.
21. _____. *The Discovery of the Orgone.* Vol. 2, *The Cancer Biopathy.* New York: Orgone Institute Press, 1948.
22. Van Doren, Carl. *Benjamin Franklin.* New York: The Viking Press, 1938.
23. Walmsley, D. M. *Anton Mesmer.* London: Robert Hale, 1967.
24. Wydenbruck, Nora. *Doctor Mesmer, an Historical Study.* London: John Westhouse, 1947.

Recommended Reading on The Life Energy

by Wilhelm Reich, M.D. Published by Farrar, Straus & Giroux, New York:
Character Analysis, 3rd edition
Function of the Orgasm, 2nd edition
The Cancer Biopathy
The Sexual Revolution
The Murder of Christ: The Emotional Plague of Mankind
Selected Writings
Reich Speaks of Freud
Ether, God and Devil
Cosmic Superimposition

Elsworth F. Baker. *Man in the Trap.* New York: Macmillan Co., 1967.
The Journal of Orgonomy, Orgonomic Publications, Inc., Box 565, Ansonia Station, New York, N.Y. 10023.
Ola Raknes. *Wilhelm Reich and Orgonomy.* New York: St. Martin's, 1970.
Peter Reich. *A Book of Dreams.* New York: Harper & Row, 1973.

INDEX

219

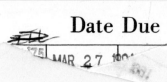